THE
FAMILY
WELLNESS
GUIDE

From Mother Earth with Love

TARA FELLNER

Illustrations by Becky Ankeny

JOURNEY EDITIONS

Boston ~ Tokyo

*This book is dedicated to my grandmother, Flora Brabender,
and my mother, Marlene Fellner, who, by example, taught kindness,
a love of gardening, and compassion for all living things.*

First published in 1998 by Journey Editions, an imprint of Periplus Editions (HK) Ltd., with
editorial offices at 153 Milk Street, Boston, Massachusetts 02109.

Warning:
The purpose of this book is to educate. It is sold with the understanding that the author and
Tuttle Publishing shall have neither liability nor responsibility for any injury caused or alleged to
be caused directly or indirectly by the information contained in this book. The adoption and
application of the material offered in this book is at the reader's discretion and sole responsibility.
While every effort has been made to ensure its accuracy, the book's contents should not be con-
strued as medical advice. Each person's health needs are unique. To obtain recommendations
appropriate to your particular situation, please consult a qualified health care provider.

Library of Congress Cataloging-in-Publication Data

Fellner, Tara.
    The family wellness guide : from mother earth with love / by Tara
Fellner.
      p.   cm.
    Includes bibliographical references and index.
    ISBN 1-885203-62-4
    1. Family—health and hygiene. 2. Holistic medicine. I. Title.
RA418.5.F3F45   1998
   613—dc21

97-48325
CIP

Distributed by

USA
Charles E. Tuttle Co., Inc.
RR 1 Box 231-5
North Clarendon, VT 05759
Tel.: (802) 773-8930
Fax.: (802) 773-6993

Japan
Tuttle Shokai Ltd.
1-21-13, Seki
Tama-ku, Kawasaki-shi
Kanagawa-ken 214, Japan
Tel.: (044) 833-0225
Fax.: (044) 822-0413

Southeast Asia
Berkeley Books Pte. Ltd.
5 Little Road #08-01
Singapore 536983
Tel.: (65) 280-3320
Fax.: (65) 280-6290

First edition
07 06 05 04 03 02 01 00 99 98 10 9 8 7 6 5 4 3 2 1

Design by Learning Arts
Cover Design by Jill A. Feron
Cover Illustrations by Becky Ankeny
Printed in the United States of America

CONTENTS

ccording to the World Health Organization, 80 percent of the people on our planet currently entrust their health care to natural remedies and traditional practitioners. Our Mother Earth provides not only the basic food, water, and shelter we need to survive, but also wonderful medicinal herbs, plants, and flowers to comfort, soothe, and heal. This book presents just a few of the many available alternative natural remedies that can contribute to a holistically balanced state of body, mind, and spirit. I have selected modalities for their usefulness, simplicity and effectiveness, choosing those proven by personal experience. They are safe, accessible, and easy to understand. Many of them I use daily in my own home, on myself and my family.

Herbs and essential oils have been used for purposes of healing for thousands of years. Subtle medicines, such as the flower essences and homeopathics described in the following chapters, are not intended to interact directly with the body on the physical level. Yet their energetic, vibratory action mobilizes the body's own vital healing force, which can result in the alleviation of physical symptoms.

It is now twenty years since I read Peter Tompkins and Christopher Bird's groundbreaking book, *The Secret Life of Plants,* in which they presented results of experiments indicating that plants have measurable reactions to the intentions, thoughts, and feelings of human beings who interact with them. Since that time I have found many confirmations of the book's concepts and conclusions in the long-standing traditions of aboriginal cultures, in subsequent scientific experiments and in my own experience. Therefore, it is a basic assumption of this book that plants are sentient beings with feelings, intelligence, and the ability to communicate on an intuitive level with human beings.

To take this idea a step further, I have also observed that people who have a close feeling relationship with nature tend to experience the most successful results from natural healing methods. If you think about it, this makes sense. As George Washington Carver once observed, that which we love will reveal to us its secrets. I believe that when we live in loving relationship with the natural world around us, we stay in sync with nature, and are more easily influenced by her subtle healing energies.

In this respect, healing is not something we "do" to or for each other; it is an ongoing, working relationship with ourselves and the world around us. For this reason, I have included a number of stories, games, crafts, and awareness exercises designed to enhance and deepen your relationship with yourself, your family, and the natural world. To quote Jesse Jackson on this subject, "Your children need your presence more than they need your presents." Sometimes the simple act of being fully present and available for ourselves and our loved ones can be a healing experience.

There is no one answer to the question of how best to promote and maintain perfect health, no one modality that will serve every illness in every individual every time. Use a combination of intuition and pragmatism to find what works best for you and your family. Don't be afraid to mix and match modalities, to be creative and to play. Health is much more than simply the absence of disease. It's a state of being actively in touch with our own living mystery. A good life, like a good healing, always contains a few sparks of magic.

By teaching ourselves and our children to be cocreators of health on all levels, it is my hope and belief that many chronic diseases and much unnecessary suffering, both human and planetary, can be averted and that a healthy, happy, harmonious state of being can become the norm for Mother Earth and all her children.

My deep appreciation extends to Michael Kerber of Charles E. Tuttle Co., Inc., and to Ron Schultz of Learning Arts Publications for the wonderful opportunity to share this healing knowledge with other families, and to Becky Ankeny for her beautiful illustrations. Thanks also to editors Kathleen King and Sheila Berg for their care and attention to detail, which helped to clarify both the text and intention of the book, and to Terry Duffy and Glyphics for putting it all together.

I am also grateful for all my family and friends, who have so often and so graciously consented to be my guinea pigs over the years as I have experimented with the different kinds of remedies presented in this book. Special thanks to my children, Nick, Maggie, and Alice, and to Paul, for being my teachers and for accompanying me on this healing journey. Russell Means, Howard Lyman, Neil Einbund, Paul Fleiss, Lani Jeansdottir and the Meadowborn Midwives, thank you for inspiring me with the healing work you do daily.

To Mother Earth and Father Sky, Mom and Dad Haugner, Jack and Shirley Shabazian, Miguel and Edna Lucia Lopez, Maureen MacFarlane, my mother, Marlene, and all the parents who tend the sparks of hope for the future as they so lovingly nurture and sustain us, warm blessings and many thanks.

—Tara

CHAPTER ONE

EARTH AWARENESS and NATURAL HEALTH

An Overview

The earth and myself are of one mind.
The measure of the land
and the measure of our bodies are the same.

—Chief Joseph, Nez Perce (1830–1904)

O nce upon a time, healing was considered an art. The healer enhanced the canvas of human being with careful strokes from a rich palette of healing colors coaxed from living herbs and trees and flowers of the field. Body, mind, and spirit were threads interwoven in a living tapestry. Human health was viewed as a partnership with the natural world, indivisible from the sacred.

In our time, the unified worldview by which our ancestors lived has been shattered. The art of healing has been replaced by the science of medicine, from whose sterile corridors the sacred is banned. However, just as quantum physics has called into question many of our most basic assumptions about the nature of reality, recent and fascinating research is giving scientific validity to concepts integral to holistic thinking, as we shall see later in this chapter.

Most of us who are parents today were raised to believe that we should put our faith in the curative powers of the family doctor and the miracle drugs, often antibiotics, which he was likely to prescribe. In accordance with the mechanistic worldview that has dominated Western culture for the last three centuries, we were conditioned to view illness as a kind of mechanical breakdown in our physical vehicle, with the solution being something akin to auto repair: when the vehicle isn't running properly, it's taken to the mechanic (doctor) where the malfunctioning part is identified (diagnosis) and either repaired, removed, or replaced (prescription, surgery, or transplant).

But human beings are vastly more complex than even the most technologically advanced automobile. The more we learn, the more we realize how little we know about ourselves and how we function. The crucial philosophical and conceptual differences between conventional medicine and alternative or natural healing practices lie not only in the substances and methods used, but also in the importance placed on intangible, and for the most part *invisible* factors, such as consciousness, emotions, life or vital forces, and spirituality. These factors are becoming more important as conventional medicine fails to address the root causes of illness and disease.

I realized after the birth of my first child some ten years ago that there are many things directly affecting our health and the health of our children, over which we have little or no control whatsoever. This realization drove me to become actively involved with antinuclear and pro-environment causes, in an effort to have a broader and more positive influence on my son's, and subsequently my daughters', future. It quickly became evident that what was best for my children tended to benefit the planet as well.

As a result of changes we have made in our environment and way of living, human beings are on the brink of a global health crisis that transcends national boundaries and differences in ethnicity, class, age, and status. The entire human family is at risk. We are, as a species, getting sicker, more tired, and less able to fight back. The state of our health mirrors the state of our planet.

EARTH TO HUMANS *The Health Connection*

*Often in the stillness of the night, when all nature seems asleep about me,
there comes a gentle rapping at the door of my heart. I open it; and a voice
inquires, "Pokagon, what of your people? What will their future be?" My
answer is: "Mortal man has not the power to draw aside the veil of unborn
time to tell the future of his race. That gift belongs of the Divine alone.
But it is given to him to closely judge the future by the present, and the past."*

—Simon Pokagon, Potawatomie (1830–1899)

About 70 percent of the American population now lives in cities.
We cityfolk spend an inordinate amount of time in boxes of our
own choice or design. Houses, apartments, and buildings are then
subdivided into rooms, or smaller boxes. To travel from one box
to the next, we get into a box with wheels. Most of us are born in
boxes within boxes, and, at the end of our lives, we are buried in
them. Boxes enclose and define space for us, making an otherwise
limitless reality a bit more manageable and less threatening on a
day-to-day basis. We take up a lot of space inside our boxes. We
appear proportionately larger and more important. But we pay a
price for the maintenance of this illusion. Our boxes separate us,
both physically and conceptually, from the vast and intricate web
of life in the natural world. We have lost, almost entirely, a sense
of perspective regarding our place within the context of the planet
upon which we've evolved. To many people, the Earth is nothing
more than a convenient storehouse from which we can take the
stuff we need to fill up our boxes endlessly. We continue our
consumerist behavior, regardless of dwindling resources and
abundant warnings that our activities cannot be sustained.

Mitakuye oyasin, the Sioux say. "We are all related." We can
only be as healthy as our environment. The time has come for us
to see our boxes and boundaries for the artificial constructs they
really are. Our responsibilities as human beings extend far beyond
the boundaries we draw on maps. Individual choices can have far-
reaching consequences. As the American Indian activist Russell
Means has said, "We have the freedom to be responsible." If we
continue to pump our planet full of poisons and destroy her
oxygen-producing forests, we cannot expect the Earth to be able
to sustain life indefinitely as we know it.

What we do to the Earth we eventually do to ourselves. The consequences of our actions come full circle, and there are now countless examples to illustrate this fact. DDT, an insecticide widely sprayed throughout the world to control mosquitoes and other insects, has reappeared as an ingredient in mother's breast milk and is also found stored in the fatty tissues of Eskimos living in the Arctic Circle, where insecticides and pesticides have never been used. PCBs, or polychlorinated biphenyls—industrial chemicals that were banned in this country in 1978 and that have been found to have adverse effects on neurological development, especially in babies and children—are still present in our environment and food supply twenty years later and will be with us for centuries to come. Clusters of cancer have shown up in populations living downwind from nuclear reactors. One in four Americans, including ten million children under the age of twelve, currently lives within four miles of a toxic waste dump.[1] Truly clean, fresh air and water are now virtually impossible to find.

Traces of man-made chemicals can now be found in all humans and animals.[2] In this century, particularly following World War II, hundreds of thousands of chemicals have been developed. Some seventy thousand synthetic chemicals are currently in use, with more than a thousand new ones being developed every year. The amount of synthetic chemicals produced has seen an exponential increase, from 1.3 billion pounds in 1940 to an incredible 320 billion pounds in 1980. The consequences to human and planetary health are only beginning to be glimpsed, as environmental contaminants are implicated in a wide variety of health problems and chronic conditions. Fifty-one synthetic chemicals, a large group that includes hundreds of heavily used PCBs, furans, and dioxins, are now classified as endocrine disrupters, which in even the most minuscule concentrations can interfere with hormonal processes that affect health and human potential. Pesticide use has been linked with increasing incidences of childhood leukemia, breast cancer, infertility, and attention deficit hyperactivity disorder (ADHD).[3] The risks to our children are profound. Noting the ubiquitous presence of chemicals in our environment, Atlanta pediatrician and allergy specialist Dr. Stephen B. Edelson has observed, "It is no wonder that our children are the sickest the world has ever seen in the history of the human species."[4]

The poisoning of our children begins before birth. The growing fetus is particularly vulnerable to damage from environmental contaminants. Many chemicals and toxic agents present in the environment, such as lead, methylmercury, ethanol, and nicotine, can cross the placenta and damage the fetus. Even extremely low levels of these chemicals can have disastrous effects. A 1990 study reported in the *Journal of Pediatrics* has shown that in utero exposure to pollutants present in our environment and food supply, such as PCBs, are linked to lower intelligence scores, poor memory, and reduced attention span.[5]

For all the benefits breastfeeding bestows on the newborn, mother's milk is now part chemical cocktail. Because of the high fat content of breast milk, chemicals that tend to be stored in fatty tissues are found there, including DDT, PCBs, lead, and mercury. The deleterious effects of these dangerous chemicals reach far beyond the location from which they are applied or used. Due to global patterns of air currents, toxic pollutants are carried northward, where cooler temperatures cause them to condense and fall into soil and water. Fish and animals such as whales, seals, sea birds, and polar bears concentrate these chemicals in their tissues. The nature-centered lifestyle of indigenous northern peoples, who depend on the poisoned creatures for food, paradoxically exposes them to the toxic fallout of industrialization. Indigenous women in the extreme northern reaches of Canada's Hudson Bay carry three and a half times more PCBs in their breastmilk than women in industrialized areas.[6] Gerald Antoine, Grand Chief of the Deh-Cho First Nations in the Northwest Territories, puts it succinctly: "We're not the ones polluting the environment, but we are the ones who have to live with the effects." On South Baffin Island, Inuit women have stopped breastfeeding their babies in an effort to halt the sharp increase in ear infections, illness, and developmental disorders that children are suffering there.[7]

Yet breastmilk is still the ideal food for most infants, containing many growth- and immune-enhancing ingredients that cannot be duplicated, as well as the appropriate balance of nutrients.[8] Breastmilk contains about 5 percent protein, as opposed to cow's milk, which contains about 15 percent. Apart from newly discovered health risks associated with a too-high protein diet, we now know that a mother who starts her baby on cow's milk must also take into account the effects of antibiotics and growth hormones used on dairy herds.

Recombinant bovine growth hormone, or rBGH, is a controversial product made by Monsanto, the same giant chemical company that created Agent Orange. Subsequently renamed "bovine somatotropin," or BST, also known as BGH, or bovine growth hormone, and marketed under the trade name Posilac, it is the first of a planned line of genetically engineered products from Monsanto. Because it is impossible to detect, and labeling for the use of rBGH is not required by the FDA, the only way to be certain that milk is free of this hormone is through labeling on the carton that notes its absence. Despite Monsanto's legal battle against such labeling, the consumer's right to know was recently upheld in an Illinois court. Along with detrimental effects on the health of cows treated with rBGH, there is also concern that the use of rBGH causes milk to have increased levels of IGF-1, an insulin-like growth factor that is not broken down in the pasteurization process, and which has been linked to breast and colon cancer.[9]

A mother who chooses bottle feeding of infant formula has to consider the potential health risks of phthalate contamination, especially if the child is male. Phthalates, a by-product of the plastics industry, have been implicated in declining sperm counts in men and undescended testicles in boys who are exposed to them in the first weeks of life.[10] Pesticide contamination in tap water can also find its way into infant formula, especially for families in the Midwest, where a recent study estimates that 10 million people in 374 communities across twelve states have been exposed to weed killers and pesticides in their drinking water for years. A single glass of water taken from a tap in Williamsburg, Ohio, a suburb of Cincinnati, was found to contain ten different pesticides.[11] According to Richard Wiles of the Environmental Working Group, "At least fifty-seven thousand infants in the Midwest drink formula each year that is contaminated with atrazine and other cancer-causing weed killers."[12] What a sad state of affairs when a mother's choice is not whether to poison her newborn but how, and to what degree. Raising a healthy baby can be an extremely complex challenge in today's toxic world, requiring greater ingenuity and awareness on the part of parents than ever before.

Just after birth, an infant's nervous, respiratory, reproductive, and immune systems are not yet fully developed. As cells rapidly multiply and organs develop during those crucial early years, a child is especially vulnerable to environmental hazards. Babies and children breathe more rapidly and thus take in more air, have higher metabolic rates, and take in more food and liquid proportionate to their size than do adults. Being closer to the ground, they get more exposure to toxins found in dust, soil, and rugs as well as low-lying vapors in pesticides or radon. Hand-to-mouth behavior and time spent playing outdoors are also factors. Despite abundant research on the physiological and behavioral differences between children and adults, most federal environmental regulations are based solely on data from adults.

Because children consume more fruits, vegetables, and juices than adults, their ingestion of pesticides needs to be a matter of much more focused concern. Recently the National Academy of Sciences reported that some pesticides may interfere with immune, respiratory, and neurological functions in children and that chronic exposure, even on a low level such as may occur through daily activity and diet, can be associated with cancer, neurobehavioral impairment, and immune dysfunction.[13]

Yet pesticide use is on the rise. While industrial toxic emissions have gone down 44 percent since 1988,[14] the worldwide pesticide market is expanding for the third year in a row, having increased by another 4 percent in 1996.[15] The marketing of these poisons is big business, accounting for more than $30 billion in sales annually.[16] One third of the pesticides used on the planet are applied here in North America. In the state of California, which has led the nation in the development of progressive regulation and disclosure guidelines for pesticide use, the application of such chemicals actually increased 31 percent between 1991 and 1995, while the use of carcinogenic pesticides in the state rose an alarming 129 percent.[17] In 1991, 70 million pounds of consumer pesticides were sold nationwide, accounting for about 6 percent of total pesticide use.[18] According to an EPA survey, 85 percent of American households have at least one pesticide stored in the home, often within the reach of children. Most home users take no safety precautions, and 40 percent of those surveyed in the state of California, where three quarters of families apply pesticides in their homes and gardens, failed to read or understand the label.[19] Given that five of the fifteen most common home-use pesticides can inhibit the activity of an enzyme that is critical to normal nervous system function, and that one fifth of the total volume of pesticides used in lawn and garden applications are classified as potential carcinogens by the EPA, such lack of awareness exposes children to unconscionable risk.[20]

However, home pesticide use represents only a small fraction of possible exposure to chemicals in the environment. In 1994, American industries reported releasing more than 2 billion pounds of toxic substances into the earth, air, and water. The Office of Technological Assessment estimates that due to faulty reporting procedures, the actual amount may be up to twenty times more.[21] Nonetheless, this enormous amount represents less than half the amount of yearly pollution that industry was releasing prior to the congressionally mandated Toxic Release Inventory Act passed in 1988. Despite numerous health risks associated with exposure to pollution, until recently the average American has not had the right to know about toxic releases from smokestacks, pipelines, and other sources within his or her own community. Ninety-five percent of industrial toxic pollution being released into the environment currently does not require notification or disclosure to the general public. You can support your right to know about toxic chemicals in your community environment by calling or writing to your representative regarding HR 1636, the Children's Environmental Protection and Right-to-Know Act, currently being considered in the House of Representatives.

Ironically, it now appears that all this poisoning of ourselves and our planet with pesticides and chemicals has come to naught. When health effects to farmers and farmworkers are factored in, pesticides cannot even be shown to have increased productivity. In addition, simpler life-forms are able to adapt fairly quickly to threats to their existence. Over the course of forty-five years, 440 insect and mite species have developed genetic resistance to pesticide use. There are now seventeen species of insects that no known pesticide can kill. Over the course of twenty years, forty-eight weed species have developed resistance to herbicides.

Human evolution, however, proceeds at a slower pace. The chemical poisons we have created may well be extinguishing our future as a species, as Rachel Carson predicted more than thirty years ago in her book *Silent Spring*.[22] Seventeen percent of American couples, almost one in five, are infertile.[23] According to data from the Centers for Disease Control (CDC), pollutants and toxins have taken their place as a leading cause of death among Americans, ranking just below lifestyle-related diseases and infectious agents.[24] Not only do our environmental standards fail to take our children into account; there is very little data available or research being done on the cumulative or synergistic effects of the wide variety of health threats to which children are exposed.

Along with poisoning our food and water, we have also compromised the quality of the air we and our children breathe. Of the billions of pounds of toxic pollutants released by American industry each year, 69 percent goes into the atmosphere in the form of air pollution,[25] with attendant health costs estimated by the CDC at over $40 billion.[26] That works out to about $20 in health care costs for each pound of air pollution. According to the Natural Resources Defense Council, sixty-four thousand people die prematurely each year from cardiopulmonary causes linked to particulate air pollution.[27] Children, who spend more time outdoors and whose defenses are not fully mature, are particularly vulnerable to airborne pollution, suffering cellular damage, reduced lung function, increased susceptibility to respiratory illness, and chronic lung disease.[28] In southern California, 90 percent of children under the age of fourteen live in areas that fail to meet state and federal air quality standards. Chicago, Houston, and Philadelphia are other American cities in which children are at risk from the air they breathe.

Almost 15 million Americans were suffering from asthma in 1994, an alarming increase of 74 percent since 1984. The severity of asthma attacks has intensified as well, with fatal attacks increasing by 46 percent in the 1980s.[29] Here, too, is an instance in which the price of industrialization is being paid with the suffering of innocents. Most of the increase in asthma cases and fatal asthmatic attack is occurring among children. More than 4 million children in the United States currently have asthma.[30] According to Dr. Ann Woolcock of the University of Sydney, "There is no country in the world where studies have been done that has not had an increase in childhood asthma in the last ten years."[31] Diet, overuse of antibiotics, and air pollution have all been implicated as contributing factors. Daycare is also related to the increase. Children in daycare are exposed to more illnesses from colds and flu by coming into daily contact with more children than they otherwise would, growing up at home. Viral infections are known to trigger asthma and are a factor in 80 percent of children hospitalized for severe asthma attacks.[32]

The quality of the air we breathe is being eroded not only by pollution, but by global deforestation, which continues to progress at an alarming rate. The effects on our planet and on human health due to the loss of our rain forests are incalculable. Already, the air in our world is said to have 30 percent less oxygen than did the air our prehistoric ancestors breathed.[33] Yet every second, two and a half acres of irreplaceable rain forest are destroyed, adding up to more than 78 million acres per year, an area greater than the size of Poland.[34] Three-quarters of this rain forest destruction is done by burning, which releases billions of tons of carbon dioxide into the atmosphere and accounts for 25 percent of global carbon dioxide emissions, a significant factor in global warming.[35] In 1990 alone, more than 40 million acres were deforested, while only slightly more than 2 million were being planted.[36]

The mere planting of trees cannot offset the destruction of our rain forests, that, while accounting for only a tiny fraction of the Earth's surface, are home to *half* the species on our planet. Every day, 137 species disappear, adding up to fifty thousand extinctions each year. Seventy percent of plants currently found to be active against cancer grow only in the rain forest. The Amazon rain forest alone produces 20 percent of the world's oxygen. Two thirds of the available fresh water on Earth is found in the Amazon Basin. Twenty years ago, 14 percent of our planet's land area was still covered with rain forest. Since then, more than 1 million species have disappeared, as forested areas have dwindled to less than 7 percent.[37] At the current rate of deforestation, the rain forest could disappear within our lifetime. This is unthinkable. What will our children and grandchildren breathe?

Our actions today determine the quality of life and health for our children tomorrow. We must consider the consequences of each and every decision we make. What we buy, where it comes from, how it is produced, all will affect our children and grandchildren in the very near future. It's up to us to be aware of the impact of our choices and to make our voices heard.

HUMAN HEALTH *What the Future Holds*

The ultimate cause of human disease is the consequence of our transgression of the universal laws of life.

—Paracelsus (1493–1541), fifteenth-century physician and alchemist

According to the U.S. Centers for Disease Control, "New infections are emerging, diseases thought to be under control are returning, and many dangerous microorganisms survive drugs that used to kill them." [38] As an example, *Staphylococcus aureus,* a common cause of infections contracted in hospitals, is highly and increasingly resistant to antibiotic treatment, as is *Streptococcus pneumoniae,* a major cause of bacterial pneumonia. A 1992 article in *Science* magazine notes that in 1940, pneumococcal pneumonia could be cured in four days using 40,000 units of penicillin. Half a century later, 24 million units of penicillin per day would not be enough to prevent death from this disease. New or growing drug resistance has also been discovered recently in the organisms that cause malaria, tuberculosis, gonorrhea, meningitis, and ear infections. The latter is particularly disturbing in light of the fact that childhood ear infections are the leading cause of visits to the pediatrician. Parents brought children in for 24 million office visits related to ear infections during 1990 alone, an increase of 150 percent since 1975. [39] More than a third of the strains of *Haemophilus influenzae,* a common bacterium associated with ear infections and sinusitis, are currently resistant to ampicillin, the antibiotic drug most commonly used to combat it. [40] A recent study released by the World Health Organization also predicts the global spread of new strains of antibiotic-resistant tuberculosis. One of the study's participants, Dr. Michael Iseman of the University of Colorado, states, "The world again faces the specter of incurable tuberculosis." He adds, "This is a creation of man, not nature." [41]

The implications of untreatable strains of infectious agents are sobering, if not downright frightening. According to Laurie Garrett, Pulitzer-Prize-winning journalist and author of *The Coming Plague: Newly Emerging Diseases in a World Out of Balance,* hospitals in New York are currently being monitored for the development of resistant strains of *Staphylococcus* or *Streptococcus* bacteria. [42] Vancomycin is the last antibiotic defense against these common bacteria, which can be found in the air and on surfaces wherever people live in close contact with one another. These bacteria cause a wide variety of illnesses including strep throat, ear infections, rheumatic fever, gangrene, and encephalitis. If untreatable strains should develop, we will live in a world in which strep throat proves to be a fatal illness once again. Such a development would be especially dangerous for those increasing numbers of children and adults with lowered immunity. Those who have no health insurance and little access to health care are also vulnerable. Of Americans whose household income is less than $25,000 per year, more than a third currently have no health coverage, and the situation is not improving.[43]

In addition to the new resistant "super germs," we continually hear about apparently new diseases: toxic shock syndrome, Legionnaire's disease, Lyme disease, hepatitis C, and hantavirus, to name a few. Cryptosporidiosis, caused by an intestinal parasite, affected almost half a million people in Milwaukee, Wisconsin, in 1993 when it contaminated tap water. Over four thousand people were hospitalized.[44] E. coli bacteria in fast-food hamburgers killed four children in 1993 and sickened more than six hundred people in several states.[45]

What is causing the surge in virulent disease? Global warming and ozone depletion are implicated. With warmer temperatures, disease-carrying insects venture to higher altitudes and latitudes, such as the malaria carrying mosquito which is now found as far north as Chicago. Along with skin cancer and damage to the eyes, ozone depletion is also linked to immunosuppression, a condition that makes it easier for diseases to take hold.[46] Increasing global traffic also contributes to the problem: familiar diseases once thought under control such as diphtheria, pertussis, yellow and Dengue fever are spread by travelers who crisscross the continents. Cholera was an uninvited guest aboard an international flight that arrived last year in California, causing seventy-five people to become ill and one to die.[47] Weather can also be a factor. Cases of cholera appeared in the suburbs of Acapulco, Mexico, recently due to sanitary problems occurring in the wake of Hurricane Paulina.[48]

One of the most alarming of the new diseases is "mad cow disease," or bovine spongiform encephalopathy (BSE), which was first diagnosed in Great Britain in 1986. Cases have also been confirmed in Ireland, France, Portugal, and Switzerland.[49] BSE is a fatal neurodegenerative disease occurring in cattle, and it is believed to be caused by an infectious protein known as a "prion," for the discovery of which Dr. Stanley Prusiner won the Nobel Prize this year. A biologically bizarre entity that is neither a virus nor a bacteria and has no detectable RNA or DNA, the prion is not destroyed by cooking, canning, freezing, burning, or pickling in formaldehyde. Prion diseases evoke no immune response and can have a long incubation period. In cattle, the incubation period for BSE is estimated at two to eight years, during which time the animal may exhibit no symptoms.[50] When the disease is activated, it quickly attacks and eats away at brain tissue, creating sponge-like perforations. There is currently no test available to detect the presence of BSE in living cattle. A diagnosis can be made with certainty only by autopsy examination of the brain of an animal that has died of the disease.

In the late 1980s, the British government predicted there would be no more than twenty thousand cases of BSE in their beef and dairy cattle. As of 1996, there were one hundred sixty thousand lab-confirmed cases with a thousand new cases being reported every week.[51] The epidemic coincides with what the World Health Organization euphemistically describes as the "recycling of affected bovine material back to cattle."[52] In other words, cows, whom nature created as herbivores, were being fed the remains of other cows who were infected with the disease, and became infected themselves. Through the process known as "rendering," carcasses and waste meat products are melted down into protein that is then used in pet food, poultry, pig, beef, and dairy cow feed, cosmetics, nutritional supplements, and medicines. If an animal infected with BSE is rendered, the disease can be passed to another animal who consumes as little as one teaspoon of feed from it.[53]

In 1997, new cases of BSE are still being reported in cattle in Great Britain at a rate of about one hundred new cases per week, despite the fact that the feeding practice many have referred to as "cow cannibalism" has been formally banned there since July of 1988.[54] In August of 1997 a similar formal ban on feeding ruminant protein to ruminants was implemented in the United States by the USDA and FDA.

Transmissible spongiform encephalopathies, or TSE's, occur in a number of species, including sheep, goats, cats, minks, deer, and elk. The human version of TSE, known as Creutzfeldt-Jakob disease, or CJD, has been known to occur rarely throughout the world, almost exclusively in older people, at a rate of about one per million. However, concurrent with the BSE epidemic, a new variation of Creutzfeldt-Jakob disease began to appear in Great Britain known as nvCJD. What is disturbing and different about this new variant is that it has affected younger people, in their teens to thirties. Certain aspects of the variant disease resemble

BSE more than CJD. A recent study indicates that the causative agents of BSE and nvCJD are indeed the same and are distinct from other forms of CJD in humans, with a biochemical signature that matches prions examined in mice and monkeys experimentally infected with BSE.[55]

The fact that the infectious agent for BSE, present in the brain, spine, and retinas of infected cattle, can cross to other species implies tragic consequences for those who have consumed infected beef.[56] The British government has acknowledged that beef infected with BSE was the likely cause of death for twenty-one British young people who have died so far of the new variant of CJD.[57] Because of difficulties diagnosing the disease and an incubation period in humans that may be as long as thirty years, it is impossible at this point to guess how many people are actually infected with the nvCJD. The *British Medical Journal* estimates that the number of human beings exposed to BSE will reach more than 34 million. The Spongiform Encephalopathy Advisory Committee stated in 1996 that it may take five to ten years to determine whether the incidence rate in humans will parallel the incidence of BSE.[58] If it does, according to Dr. Richard Lacey, a Leeds University microbiologist, the better part of a whole generation of people may die.[59]

The new variant of CJD has also been reported in France and Germany. Here in the United States, a twenty-four-year-old woman in New York is believed to have contracted the disease from British beef cutlets she received as a gift.[60] Thirteen tons of British meat and bone meal were imported into this country before such products were banned in 1989.

Americans have the highest per capita beef consumption in the world. Our cattle industry accounts for the lion's share of our agricultural economy, bringing in about $150 billion a year from 100 million cattle. There is speculation that BSE is and has been present in United States beef for some time, and may be related to what is referred to in this country as "downer" cow syndrome, in which cattle come down with a disease that causes them to stagger and fall over. In 1985, minks in Wisconsin who had been fed sick "downer" dairy cows began to die of spongiform encephalopathy. A USDA internal document from 1991 stated: "There is speculation . . . that a spongiform encephalopathy agent is present in the US cattle population."[61] This possibility was confirmed by the work of University of Wisconsin virologist Richard Marsh, who drew attention to the issue prior to his death in March of 1997. Another USDA document noted that "the mere perception that BSE might exist in the United States could have devastating effects on our domestic market for beef and dairy products." [62] There is speculation that prions may build up in the system over time, and that repeated exposure to the infectious agent for BSE may increase the likelihood of contracting spongiform encephalopathy.

Tim Lang, professor of food policy at Thames Valley University in the United Kingdom, describes the BSE epidemic as follows: "We are in a mass experiment that is killing us. We have interfered with the whole process of nature, and what is now happening is one of our worst nightmares." [63]

Is our public health care system prepared to protect us from all this? Not according to the CDC. They observe that "current systems for keeping track of infectious diseases here and abroad cannot meet the threat of emerging infections. The nation's early warning system for infectious diseases . . . is in disarray. Many foodborne and waterborne disease outbreaks go unrecognized or are detected late. Global disease surveillance is rudimentary." [64]

In other words, we're going to have to take care of ourselves. According to Howard F. Lyman, president of the International Vegetarian Union, simply by eliminating animal products from our diets we can cut the amount of carcinogens we ingest by more than 90 percent. A fourth-generation rancher and feed-lot operator from Montana who lectures worldwide, Mr. Lyman is among those being sued for remarks made on a now-famous episode of the *Oprah Winfrey Show* in which BSE and the realities of the meat industry were vigorously discussed.

Support natural, earth-friendly, organic, and sustainable practices with your dietary choices. What you and your family choose to eat and where it comes from are increasingly a matter of life and death.

NATURAL HEALING

The art of healing comes from Nature and not from the physician.

—Paracelsus

Unlike conventional medicine, which focuses on the blanket treatment of symptoms and disease overall, natural healing takes its inquiry beyond the manifestation of illness to consider the unwell person as an individual and whole being. Whereas allopathic medicine since the mid-nineteenth century has focused on the treatment of tangible, physical symptoms and the detection and eradication of their causative agents ("germ theory"), alternative forms of medicine are more concerned with the balanced and harmonious interaction of body, mind, and spirit. In addition, natural healing methods assume that the body is fully capable of healing itself once proper conditions for its optimal functioning are reestablished. Certain natural organic substances are assumed to be most compatible with this process.

In the allopathic approach to medicine, the role of the individual in maintaining his or her own health is greatly overshadowed by surgeons and physicians seen to be endowed with miraculous, almost godlike powers of life and death. In cases of severe trauma and advanced pathology, they can save limbs, remove tumors, and transplant diseased or worn-out organs. In the laboratory, the medical/scientific priesthood explores the mysteries of our very being, altering cell structure and DNA, even engineering in a test tube the moment at which life begins. Sophisticated devices such as EEGs, EKGs, MRIs, X rays, and ultrasound allow them to see into us with unprecedented accuracy and clarity. Pharmaceutical drugs manipulate brain and body chemistry and make annoying, unsightly, or painful symptoms seem to go away.

But all too often the allopathic patient trades one set of symptoms for a new, "iatrogenic disease," an additional set of problems caused by the drug or treatment prescribed. One illness may be "cured," but another has taken its place. As an extreme example of this commonly accepted phenomenon of allopathic side effects, Burton Goldberg's excellent *Alternative Medicine* reports that in this country, 0.44% of hospitalized patients have fatal reactions to drug use, resulting in more than 350 deaths every day. If the use of herbs and natural remedies were resulting in this many fatalities, all such products would be banned from the marketplace. Often a single fatal reaction is sufficient cause to remove an herb or supplement from health food store shelves.

While conventional medicine excels in miraculous and dramatic rescues, it has failed utterly to provide us with the day-to-day tools we need to maintain a healthy physiological balance and to prevent disease before it has taken root. All too often there is no true "healing" taking place, only a superficial "cure" for one set of symptoms that merely displaces illness in another form to a different part of the body. As more and more invasive methods of attempted treatment are employed, ranging from antibiotics to major surgery, the basic health of the body can be seriously undermined.

According to the principles of natural healing, true health encompasses much more than adequate bodily function. The healthiness of an individual's relationships, work patterns, spirituality, and habitual thoughts and feelings is also considered. Adverse symptoms in any of these areas are viewed as an attempt by the self to communicate an imbalance or need that must be addressed. Thus illness itself is a healer, drawing our attention to those areas in our lives that need perfecting. Some of those who are and have been active within the alternative healing movement, such as Alice Steadman (author of *Who's the Matter with Me?*), Louise Hay (*You Can Heal Your Life*), and Thorwald Dethlefson (*The Healing Power of Illness*), have taken this a step further and categorized physical symptoms according to the emotional, psychological, or behavioral imbalances they may represent.

Fundamental to an understanding of natural healing is acceptance of the idea that there is a vital force within each one of us that sustains life and health. In Western metaphysical traditions, this concept corresponds to the theoretical existence of the "etheric double," or health aura, a subtle body of invisible energy that coexists with and interpenetrates the physical body, serving as a kind of intermediary between consciousness and physical being. Until now, subtle energies were not scientifically verifiable because equipment capable of measuring them did not exist. But quantum theory seems to be closing the gap between science and metaphysics. Scientific verification of the existence of the health aura may have been recently discovered by Vladimir Poponin, a Russian quantum physicist and world-renowned researcher in the cutting-edge field of quantum biology.

In a 1992 study conducted at the Russian Academy of Sciences, a DNA sample was placed in a laser photon correlation spectrometer (LPCS). Measurements were taken inside the LPCS before and after the DNA was placed inside. According to Dr. Poponin, "When the DNA is removed from the scattering chamber, one anticipates that the autocorrelation function will be the same as before the DNA was placed in the scattering chamber." No one was more surprised than the researchers when this was not the case. After the DNA was physically removed from the chamber, something left behind an energetic imprint that was measurably different. Puzzled, the researchers repeated the experiment numerous times, each time getting similar results. "We were forced to accept the working hypothesis that some new field structure is being excited from the physical vacuum," Dr. Poponin states, noting that "as long as the space in the scattering chamber is not disturbed, we are able to measure this effect for long periods of time. In several cases we have observed it for up to a month." What is this subtle energy residue? Dr. Poponin suggests that his discovery, which he refers to as "the DNA Phantom Effect" may explain such things as the phantom limb, in which pains or sensations persist after a limb has been amputated, as well as the success of certain alternative healing modalities.[65]

We can inhibit or strengthen our vital force depending on the choices and decisions we make. Our lifestyles, what we put into our bodies, what we think and feel, and the intensity of our will to live all determine how brightly this inner flame burns. Poor lifestyle choices, toxic substances, and negative emotions erode our vitality and depress immune function. Good nutrition, a healthy environment, positive emotions, loving relationships, and a sense of meaning and spiritual connection enhance the life force and consequently raise the effectiveness of our body's defenses.

Maintenance of a healthy vital force is especially important for parents of young children. According to Eastern healing traditions, the energy that vitalizes the body originates in the center and flows outward to the extremities through invisible channels paralleling the nervous system. Children are born with incomplete energy channels, causing them to draw heavily on the energy of their parents to fuel continued growth and development and to recover from illnesses when they occur. Children may also, as they absorb vital energy from their mothers or fathers, consciously or unconsciously internalize unresolved problems or conflicts originating within their parents or the parents' relationship, which can result in physical, emotional, or mental health problems.

As even those who are well known for their healing abilities will tell you, one person cannot really heal another. Healing is an intensely personal, inner process of repair, a chosen movement away from disease and toward health. At its most basic, it is a renewed connection with, and commitment to, the profound and mysterious force that sustains all of life. Substances such as herbs, essential oils, homeopathic remedies, and flower essences are believed to hold vibratory patterns necessary to redirect the flow of energy within the sick or diseased person. However, the intention and love with which such substances are administered are just as important as the substances themselves.

Natural remedies support the body's own healing process, rather than eclipse or override it. They are especially helpful in achieving and maintaining balance between body, mind, and spirit. On the physiological, or "body" level, the most basic building block of natural health is a strong immune system.

THE IMMUNE SYSTEM *How It Works*

The purpose of our immune system is to recognize things that do not belong in the body and to get rid of them. These foreign invaders may include viruses, bacteria, fungi, or substances such as heavy metals and environmental pollutants. As immune cells circulate through the bloodstream, they also endeavor to keep arteries clear.

The thymus is the immune system's "command center." This gland is relatively large in an infant but begins to shrink by the age of eight or ten years, until it is about the size of a thumb in an adult. T cells, produced in the thymus, coordinate the activities and production of lymphocytes in response to infection. Typically, a patient with an immune dysfunction, such as AIDS, will have an abnormal T cell ratio, or count.

The lymphatic system consists of the lymph nodes, liver, bone marrow, and spleen. Immune cells are produced in bone marrow, the lymph nodes, tonsils, and spleen. There are basically two types of immune cells: "memory" cells, which hold the memory of specific pathogens and attack them whenever they perceive their presence, and "effector" cells, which attack any and all invaders. Lymph nodes often swell due to increased activity when the immune system is fighting an infection, resulting in "swollen glands" in the neck, armpits, or groin.

Immune cells start their lives as featureless "stem" cells that only later take on characteristics that differentiate them as a specific kind of cell, such as a red blood cell, which delivers oxygen to cells and carries away carbon dioxide, or one of five types of white blood cells, also known as leukocytes, which police the body through the circulatory system. Immunostimulant herbs and essential oils, which will be described in depth in later chapters, stimulate production of stem cells in the spleen, marrow, and lymph tissue and then speed up their development into active immune cells.

Immunostimulants also enhance the activity of macrophages and lymphocytes. Macrophages are the white blood cells that destroy and

The Immune System

literally eat up foreign invaders such as germs, viruses, and bacteria in a process called phagocytosis. Extract of echinacea, for example, has been shown to increase phagocytosis by 20 to 40 percent. The removal of infectious agents, waste, and debris keeps the blood and body systems clean and functioning as they should.

If we develop a disease, it means the immune system has failed to do its job. Immune function can be depressed by a variety of stressors, such as infections, pollution, junk food, and negative emotions. Conversely, proper diet, the correct balance of vitamins and minerals, and positive emotional states support immune function. Recent research also indicates that the immune system has a capacity to remember and to learn, and will respond to conditioning. In other words, intelligence is not limited to the brain. It is now being shown to exist in every cell of the body. There is no longer any clear line between body and mind.

HEALTH AND EMOTION   *The Body/Mind Connection*

A cheerful heart is good medicine, but a downcast spirit dries up the bones.

—Proverbs 17:22

It matters how you feel. In fact, how you feel on a day-to-day basis can be a matter of life and death. Emotions can have tremendous impact on health and bodily function. Fascinating new research is beginning to show how and why.

For more than twenty years, Dr. Candace Pert, former chief of brain biochemistry at the National Institutes of Health (NIH), has been studying peptides and receptors found in the limbic system, immune system, and autonomic nervous system. Her work has convinced her that these chains of amino acids, found throughout the brain and the body, are the biological basis for emotion. Among the first peptides identified in the 1970s were endorphins, shorthand for endogenous morphines, opiate-like chemicals that create a sense of pleasure and well-being.

The limbic system of the brain regulates basic drives and emotion. Within the hippocampus, part of the limbic system, Dr. Pert has found "almost every variety of peptide." Peptide receptors, which are activated when we experience or recall emotion, can also be found in organs, tissue, skin, muscle, and throughout the endocrine system. The sum total of all these peptide receptors form the peptide network, which also functions as a storehouse for emotional memory. According to Dr. Pert, "This means the emotional memory is stored in many places in the body, not just the brain." In effect, her work erases the line between body and mind.[66]

The experience of many bodyworkers, whose clients have experienced the release of sometimes deeply buried emotions during massage sessions, confirms their belief that emotional memory is stored throughout the body. Dr. Pert has observed that emotion that is not fully expressed can be stored in muscles, tissue, or organs. To reach conscious awareness, an emotion must travel through the nervous system, up the spinal cord into the higher regions of the brain. However, the brain's cortex is very picky about the information it will allow into awareness. So much is going on in the body at any given time that being fully conscious of every single neural activity would quickly create a state of overload. To prevent this from happening, the cortex sends out chemicals and impulses to repress what it perceives as unnecessary information. An emotion that does not reach conscious awareness cannot be expressed and is stored at the site at which it was successfully repressed. What effect does this have on health? Dr. Pert states, "I think there is overwhelming evidence that unexpressed emotion causes illness."

How does unexpressed emotion cause illness? Dr. Pert elaborates, "Viruses use the same receptors [as neuropeptides] to enter into a cell, and depending on how much of the natural peptide for that receptor is around, the virus will have an easier or harder time getting into the cell. So our emotional state will affect whether we'll get sick from the same loading dose of a virus."

Emotion is also gaining recognition as a key factor in memory, learning, and intelligence. We are now beginning to recognize that the idea of intelligence as "pure" reason, brain function "unclouded" by feeling or emotion, is a myth. Emotion directs human thought, particularly the higher intellectual processes such as reason, logic, and analytical thinking, not the other way around. Just as quantum physics challenges and expands our cherished ideas about the nature of physical reality, new research demonstrates that the Cartesian ideal may have been putting the cart before the horse. Descartes's search for something that cannot be doubted may have to be rephrased, from "I think, therefore I am," to "I feel, therefore I think."

Supporting the concept of a heart-centered "emotional intelligence" are the intricate and demonstrable connections between the heart and the brain. Brain and heart functions are inextricably intertwined through the sympathetic and parasympathetic nervous systems via the vagus nerves, which connect the heart, pharynx, larynx, and abdominal viscera to the brain. Physical responses to emotion can be experienced whether the emotion is occurring in the present moment, being recalled, or just vividly imagined, as any good actor can corroborate. Blushing, a racing heartbeat, a lump in the throat, or knots in the stomach experienced as part of emotional response are all evidence of the brain/heart connection.

In addition, as a 1996 study reported in the medical journal *Stroke* has shown, a trauma to the head or stroke which causes bleeding in the brain will concurrently cause life-threatening damage to the walls of the heart. Why? "Confirmation of the brain-heart connection gives us a possible explanation for these deaths," one of the Pittsburgh-based researchers states.[67]

Brain and heart are not only biochemically and neurally connected; they are electrically coupled as well. When "brain waves," patterns of electrical activity in the brain, were first recorded by the German psychiatrist Hans Berger in 1929, his work was ridiculed by other scientists. New ideas often meet with resistance. But new ideas can also take root rapidly. A short three years later, the British electrophysiologist Edgar Adrian won a Nobel Prize for demonstrating the same phenomenon. Bioelectricity is now an active field of study and research. Robert Becker, an orthopedic surgeon and author of *The Body Electric,* pioneered the use of electricity in speeding the body's healing processes. He has also shown that people under hypnosis are capable of using directed thought to create voltage changes in the body.

Most of us are familiar with the monitoring of electrical activity in the brain using the EEG, or electroencephalograph. The human heart puts out an electromagnetic field as well. Electrical impulses from the sinoatrial node, the heart's "pacemaker," initiate the muscle contractions we perceive as our "heartbeat." This pacemaking activity is regulated by the sympathetic nervous system, which speeds it up, and the parasympathetic system, which inhibits contractions, thereby slowing it down. A heartbeat produces a 2.5 watt electrical signal that reaches every cell in the body. Our thoughts and emotions influence the quality of this electrical signal, which is forty to sixty times more powerful in amplitude than that of the brain.

In a study published in the *American Journal of Cardiology* in 1995, spectral analysis of heart rate variability as recorded by electrocardiograph, or EKG readings demonstrated not only the effect of emotion on the sympathetic and parasympathetic response, but also actual differences in electrical frequency between negative and positive emotions.[68] Just as varying levels of consciousness such as alpha, beta, theta, and delta are reflected in changing brain wave patterns, different emotions register as different patterns in heart wave graphs.

Anger registers as chaotic, weak, high-frequency heart waves, while love and appreciation create orderly, low frequency, powerful waves. Results of the study additionally suggest that managing our emotions through positive redirection can reduce the effects of hypertension and heart disease, lower high blood pressure, and reduce the likelihood of sudden death from heart attack.

Exercise

How can we keep emotions from lodging in the body and causing illness? Mostly it's a matter of being more aware of ourselves. Often before we cognitively identify an emotion, we experience a change in tension somewhere in the body. If this is effectively suppressed from awareness, the emotion gets lodged there. Good indicators that unexpressed emotion has gotten "stuck" somewhere in the body are feelings of numbness, heaviness, detachment, or depression. There can be physical tension or stiffness in the part of the body where the emotion was halted in its progress toward the brain. On a mental level, we may start to feel disconnected from people and things we normally care about. Another clue is inappropriate displacement of emotion: we become irritable, critical of ourselves and others, and project the trapped emotion onto external events or those around us.

To release emotion that has been trapped in the body, try the following exercise. Sit down, relax, and disengage from all external distractions. Turn off the phone, the TV, the CD player. Just be with yourself in silence. Now, take a few deep breaths. Are there a lot of thoughts clamoring for your attention? See them as a noisy flock of birds wheeling to and fro against a dull gray sky. Beneath their squawking cries and frenetic, beating wings there is a wide, empty field, a peaceful, open space. Let the flock of bird/thoughts fly away as you quietly move your awareness into the silent, open space. Rest there for a moment. Now begin to narrow the focus of your consciousness, concentrating it into a powerful beam. Think of your awareness as a kind of searchlight, or flashlight. You're going to use it to have a look around the inside of your house, your body, that which is enclosed by your skin.

Now, take a look around. Scanning your physical body with your awareness, ask yourself, what doesn't feel right? Once you've located a place in the body that seems out of kilter, give it all your attention. Pay special attention to any words or images that may pop into your awareness. Tension in the stomach, for example, might present an image of knotted rope. You can ask yourself, what does this mean? What is tying me in knots? Listen carefully to your responses. When you have the right answer, a feeling of "rightness" will accompany it. As the causative issue comes into your awareness, you'll feel the physical tension begin to release as the trapped emotion reaches the cognitive level. You can help this process along with visualization, for example, imagining that you are gently and lovingly untying the knots. You may feel a rush of emotion, a kind of Aha! as the cortex "realizes," or allows into your reality, the trapped event. Once you've experienced it, allow any accompanying emotion to be released along with the physical tension. You may feel like releasing with tears, or exhaling the emotion with some deep, cleansing breaths.

Tensions that are very deeply lodged in the body/mind as a result of suppressed trauma or extremely painful experiences may require a combination of psychotherapy and bodywork to release fully. Rolfing, Trager work, Feldenkrais, and Alexander Technique are just a few of the types of bodywork available to facilitate deeper levels of physical and emotional release.

THE POWER OF LOVE

Love is the opening door
Love is what we came here for
No one could offer you more. . . .

—Leslie Duncan, *Love Song*

> *Love is the most powerful and still the most*
> *unknown energy of the world.*
>
> —Pierre Teilhard de Chardin

Children need love,
especially when they do not deserve it.

—Harold S. Hulbert, *A Mother's Journal*

We all need love, whether we deserve it or not. I consider love separately from emotion. While many emotions may attend the experience of loving, love itself is a powerful, intangible force that is capable of transforming the nature of being and reality as we know it. As Russian poet and novelist Boris Pasternak observed, "Compared to other feelings, love is an elemental cosmic force weaving a disguise of meekness. . . . it is not a state of mind; it is the foundation of the universe." Healing, health, respect for life, and spiritual connection are all hallmarks of the functional presence of that invisible but undeniable energy we label "love," and I await with longing the day when love is as well studied and well documented as other invisible, yet obvious and powerful energies—such as electricity, magnetism, and nuclear fission and fusion—that we have learned to tap into and channel.

Children are particularly sensitive to the presence or lack of love, which can influence their development from the moment of conception onward. Some researchers believe that the newly fertilized ovum may possess consciousness and enough awareness to choose whether or not it will continue to develop. Babies even die from lack of love, or suffer stunted growth and mental retardation. Until relatively recently, a phenomenon known as "psychosocial dwarfism," a failure-to-thrive condition manifesting as impaired mental and physical development, was believed to be caused by insufficient growth hormone from the pituitary gland. Deeper study, however, has revealed that the pituitary insufficiency is caused by a lack of love by one or both parents, usually the mother.[69]

Love between human beings is expressed by general caretaking behaviors, but most directly by touch: kissing, hugging, holding, caressing. "To be tender, loving, and caring," Ashley Montagu observes in his book *Touching: The Human Significance of the Skin*, "human beings must be tenderly loved and cared for in their earliest years, from the moment they are born. Where touching begins, there love and humanity also begin—within the first minutes following birth."

Stimulation of the skin enhances immune function, while lack of touching, especially for infants separated from their mothers, has been shown to lower lymphocyte response. The skin itself produces a substance immunochemically indistinguishable from a hormone produced in the thymus gland that is related to T cell differentiation. Again, the intricate connections among the physical body, emotion, and immune function are apparent.

Love raises endorphin levels and increases pain threshold while lowering blood pressure and lactic acid levels, produced by fatigued muscles, in the blood. Some studies showed that married men live longer and even have fewer car accidents provided their wives kiss them good-bye in the morning.[70] A Stanford study of breast cancer patients found that those involved in a loving support group lived twice as long as those who did not participate.[71] Love has been shown to improve the effectiveness of white blood cells in fighting infection. There is increasing evidence that it may even prevent heart disease. An Israeli study showed that for men who had angina, the single greatest predictor of whether they would develop further heart problems was a "no" answer to the question, "Does your wife show you her love?"[72]

Merely being in the presence of love, or watching compassion in action can have health benefits as well, as demonstrated by a famous study conducted by Harvard psychologists, in which increased levels of immunoglobulin-A were detected in the saliva of people who had watched a documentary about Mother Teresa's missionary work in India.[73] Salivary immunoglobulin A (S-IgA), an antibody found in mucous secretions, is a first-line defense against pathogens that infect the upper respiratory tract, gastrointestinal system, and urinary tract. The higher your levels of S-IgA, the less likely you are to be susceptible to upper respiratory infections such as colds, flu, or bronchitis.

A similar study reported in a 1995 issue of the *Journal of Advancement in Medicine* takes the Harvard study one step further.[74] Noting the dearth of studies exploring the effects of positive emotions on the immune system, Drs. Glen Rein, Mike Atkinson, and Rollin McCraty measured S-IgA levels in thirty people before and after experiencing emotional states of anger and compassion. Like the Harvard study, they too used the Mother Teresa documentary as an external stimulus for the care/compassion state, and a video of war scenes to evoke anger. However, in addition to the external methods, they also had their subjects self-induce the required emotional states.

Interestingly, the war video produced a wide variety of responses from participants and did not succeed in evoking a state of anger that could be sustained. All participants managed to self-induce anger by recalling situations in their own lives that made them feel angry and frustrated (more evidence of the body/mind connection). They experienced a significant increase in heart rate and mood disturbance, along with physical symptoms such as headache and muscle pain, which lasted three to six hours after the experience was over. Anger was shown to lower their immunity, decreasing S-IgA levels and keeping them low for five hours afterward.

To self-induce feelings of care and compassion, an emotional management technique called "Freeze-Frame" was taught to the participants. Using this method, attention is shifted to the physical area around the heart, and participants then focus on their feelings of care or compassion toward someone or something dear to them. This caused S-IgA levels to increase even more than they did when the subjects were watching the Mother Teresa video, as high as 240 percent in some of those studied, with elevated levels continuing for up to six hours afterward. The researchers concluded that "self-induction of a positive emotional state is more effective at stimulating S-IgA than external methods." In other words, we ourselves are most effective at creating within ourselves the kind of body/mind state that best promotes good health. (For a brief description of the Freeze-Frame technique, see the "Resource Guide.")

An article in a 1988 issue of the journal *Science*, supported with citations from no fewer than sixty-two studies, states that people who habitually maintain a loving, caring approach toward life and who have warm relationships with others have better immune response overall, live longer, recover faster, and are less likely to get sick in the first place. The level of activity of their immune system's killer cells is higher, as is their S-IgA level even when they are stressed.[75] An extensive nine-year study published in the *American Journal of Epidemiology* in 1979 also concluded that people who maintain loving social ties and relationships are more resistant to disease and live longer.[76] Conversely, negative emotional states, excessive life stress, and social withdrawal have an immunosuppressive effect, decreasing the production of lymphocytes and inhibiting natural killer cell activity as well as reducing levels of S-IgA.

Over the long run, effects of a habitually negative emotional state can manifest as diseases related to immune dysfunction, heart disease, and other chronic illnesses. Working women with children, regardless of the number of children or their marital status, are particularly at risk. A recent study conducted at Duke University indicated that the greatly increased stress load experienced by working mothers may predispose them to heart disease due to elevated activation of stress hormones which can raise blood pressure, a major risk factor for heart attack.[77] Heart disease, still the number one killer of women and men in the United States, is equated on a spiritual/emotional level with a lack of love and joy in life in Louise Hay's best-selling book *You Can Heal Your Life*.

Women are more prone to depression, being twice as likely as men to be diagnosed with this condition. One woman in five will likely experience a period of major depression during her lifetime, an illness most likely to hit her between the ages of 25 to 44. One in six depressed women commits suicide. Risk factors include single parenthood, poverty, small children in the home, and a history of depression in close family members.[78] Dysthymia, a milder form of depression characterized by ongoing symptoms of low energy or low self-esteem, can plague a woman for years before she seeks diagnosis or treatment. In a culture in which exploitation of and violence against women are commonplace events, stress, burnout, depression, and eating disorders are common female complaints.

Emotional management skills are crucial for children as they reach adolescence and are confronted with the complex challenges of approaching adulthood. The problems facing children and young people have changed drastically in the latter half of this century. Consider this: in 1940, teachers rated the top problems in American schools as students talking out of turn, chewing gum, making noise, and running in the halls. In 1990, the top teacher-rated problems were drug and alcohol abuse, pregnancy, suicide, and robbery, according to the U.S. Department of Commerce Bureau of the Census.[79] Such problems do not resolve themselves and are often carried into adulthood.

"It's a warning sign," says Mark Miringoff, director of the Institute for Innovation in Social Policy at the Fordham University Graduate Center. This institution's most recent (1994) U.S. Social Health study found our nation's social well-being at a twenty-five-year nadir, with children and young adults bearing the brunt of the downward spiral. Drug abuse, child abuse, and the high school dropout rate, representing three of the six major problems confronting Americans under the age of eighteen, are worsening. Teen suicide is now 95 percent higher than it was in 1970, with a majority of our young people admitting that they have considered taking their own lives. Eight out of ten teenagers worry about violence, guns, intoxicants, and whether or not they will be able to get a job. Seven million kids come home to an empty house or apartment after school. According to a recent Children's Defense Fund survey, 20 percent of American kids have less than ten minutes of conversation with their parents over the course of a month.

Dan Pursuit, quoted in *Meditations for New Mothers,* observes, "All children wear the sign: 'I want to be important NOW!' Many of our juvenile delinquency problems arise because nobody reads the sign." How children are guided emotionally not only influences their self-esteem and sense of well-being, but can have tremendous impact on their academic success and effectiveness in the world. Be sure to take time daily to "read the sign."

The following games foster positive emotion and interaction between parent and child and any others you may wish to include.

Heart Ball

This game teaches young children how to send and receive love and that learning to love is fun and feels good to the heart. This game is also beneficial for getting children back in the heart and happy when they have been cranky or upset. It can be played indoors by an adult and one to five children, on the floor, and requires a small ball, such as a Nerf ball.

Instructions

1. Child and adult sit about six feet apart on the floor. Both child and adult spread their legs apart so that the ball can easily be caught when rolled back and forth.

2. The adult then instructs the child on how to play the game. Adult says, "I am going to roll the ball to you and as I do, I am going to send love to you."

3. Before rolling the ball to the child, hold the ball against your heart for a moment. Breathe in and out as though you are filling the ball with love. Then before rolling the ball, say, "Here it comes. It's full of love."

4. When the child catches the ball, the adult asks, "Did you get my love?" After the child responds, say, "Now you put love in the ball and roll it back to me." Keep the game going as long as the child shows interest.

5. With children as young as two and three years old, you can suggest sending love to dad, mom, grandma, and so forth, as you roll the ball back and forth. Let the child decide who to send love to. It can sometimes expand to loving the entire world.

Secret Care Buddies

Care is a quality that sustains the loving spirit in families and schools, deepens the heart connection, and makes it easier to neutralize or overcome dislikes and disagreements. Simply said, care creates bonding. This game can be played by the whole family or by a group. The first time you play, it may be helpful to have each participant first make a list of little things or actions that make them feel cared for. However, even younger children are often surprisingly creative in this regard.

1. Bring everyone together and share the purpose of "Secret Care Buddies." Tell everyone they will play the game for one week with the goal of performing one caring act per day for their secret buddy. Encourage each player not to leave behind any obvious hints.

2. On strips of paper of equal size, write the name of each participant. Fold up the papers and place in a bowl. Each family (or group) member picks one name, keeping the identity hidden from the receiver of their caring actions. (Before folding the slips, make sure younger children can read or identify all of the names.)

3. Remind each other daily about playing the Secret Care Buddies game. In order to facilitate ideas, suggest that everyone ask their hearts in private what kind of caring actions would be possible. If younger children need help, tell them to ask someone who is not their secret buddy. When the week is over, everyone tries to guess the identity of their secret buddy. When all the names are revealed, discuss some of the secret strategies and the fun, caring acts everyone received.

(From Doc Lew Childre's *Teaching Children to Love; 80 Games and Fun Activities for Raising Balanced Children in Unbalanced Times* [Boulder Creek, Calif.: Planetary Publications, 1996]. Used with permission.)

BODY/MIND MEETS SPIRIT
Love, Meditation, and Prayer

I have found very few atheists among the parents of dying children.

—Former Surgeon General C. Everett Koop

My religion is kindness.

—Dalai Lama

All religions are, at their core, a structured attempt to penetrate and make sense of the mysteries of life and death. Most religions do this by careful cultivation, through various disciplines, of a loving state, which is seen as a kind of passport to direct experience of the divine. There are myriad shades and gradations of love and its expression, and though it can be difficult to measure or quantify, few people, spiritually minded or otherwise, will deny outright that love exists. While religion is a human-made form, spirituality is the eternal animating energy it attempts to contain. Some go so far as to equate the nature of the spiritual principle with love itself, that is, "God is Love."

What is particularly interesting about our time in human history is that we are beginning to document the effects and existence of this hitherto elusive, intangible energy with what was previously one of our most loveless tools. Science is being used to quantify and measure the existence of love and to catalog its beneficial effects. Science, in particular the new physics, is also being used to bridge the gap between Eastern and Western philosophies. Compare the results of Dr. Rein's studies utilizing the redirection of emotion using the Freeze-Frame technique with a Zen master's assertion "Zen is not in my view a philosophy or mysticism. It is simply a practice of readjustment of nervous activity. That is, it restores the distorted nervous system to its normal functioning." Methodologies are different, but the outcome is the same.

What is the difference between meditation and prayer? From my own experience, they are simply two different roads that ultimately end up in the same place. Meditation directs attention

33

inward for an experience of "at-one-ment," in which the meditator's intention is to become one with the spiritual energy permeating all existence. Prayer takes the impulse toward sacred connection and inner peace and projects it outward.

When prayer is directed with healing intention, it can have powerful effects, as a number of recent and ongoing studies demonstrate. A particularly famous one was reported in the *Southern Medical Journal* in 1988. Following a randomized double-blind protocol, Dr. Randolph C. Byrd evaluated the therapeutic effects of intercessory prayer on 393 coronary care unit patients over a period of ten months. Those who were prayed for had a significantly lower severity score, requiring less ventilatory assistance, antibiotics, and diuretics than the control group that were not prayed for.[80] When the National Institutes of Health sponsored a survey of more than two hundred fifty studies published since the nineteenth century, a positive correlation was found between the use of healing prayer and beneficial effects on people suffering from conditions as diverse as cancer, cardiovascular disease, and colitis. Dr. Harold G. Koenig, a program director at Duke University Medical Center agrees: "All the evidence says that prayer does have an impact."

Prayer benefits the person who is praying as well as the one being prayed for, by inhibiting the release of hormones and bio-chemicals associated with stress, which improves both mental and physical health in the devout. Religion has been found to correlate with lower blood pressure in men, as reported in the *Journal of Religion and Health* in 1989.[81] Going to church and belief in God has also been demonstrated to speed recovery and lessen depression among elderly women.[82] In fact, those who go to church are four times less likely to commit suicide. A twenty-six-year survey of ten thousand civil servants in Israel concluded that extremely religious Orthodox Jews were less likely to die of heart problems.[83] In an evaluation of one thousand hospital patients between the years 1987 and 1989, Duke University researchers found that those who engaged in spiritual practices, such as prayer, were better able to cope with their illness.[84]

Other experiments, such as those conducted by William Braud and Marilyn Schlitz, suggest that the directed thought processes of one person can trigger physiological changes in another person, regardless of the distance between them.[85] Prayer, which is a form of directed thought motivated and powered by loving intention, has a particular ability to project itself across time and distance to elicit a resonant response in the object of its attention. Dr. Elizabeth Targ conducted a ten-week study in 1995 that matched twenty severely ill AIDS patients with twenty faith healers of various denominations praying on their behalf. According to Dr. Targ, those praying "included Native American healers, a fundamentalist Christian, a Chi Gong master, and many people from healing training schools."[86] The results were encouraging enough to launch a more extensive study: More than one hundred AIDS patients are now being prayed for over the course of one year.[87] Grants from the NIH's new Office of Alternative and Complementary Medicine, which received $12 million in funding from Congress for 1997, are supporting a University of New Mexico study on whether the prayers of an interdenominational group can have a positive effect on alcoholics.[88]

According to a June 1996 Time/CNN poll, 82 percent of Americans believe in the healing power of prayer. Dr. Herbert Benson of Harvard Medical School, author of *The Relaxation Response,* believes that humans are genetically "wired for God" and notes that prayer affects levels of stress hormones which in turn affect immune response. On December 5, 1995, an ABC News story reported on Dr. Benson's extensive study of the effects of meditation and prayer on heart disease, cancer, fertility rates, and blood cholesterol levels. Dr. Larry Dossey describes prayer as "the best kept secret in medicine." In a 1994 interview in *Magickal Blend* magazine, Dr. Dossey notes, "There are easily one hundred thirty studies that show that if you take prayer into the laboratory under controlled situations, it does something remarkable, not just to human beings but to bacteria, fungi, germinating seeds, rats, mice, and baby gerbils." Over half of the studies demonstrated significant results that cannot be written off as mere placebo effect: "that's difficult to do considering that bacteria, fungi, and germinating seeds aren't generally considered to be susceptible to suggestion." Religious affiliation is less important than "qualities of consciousness like caring, compassion, empathy, and love. That's what seems to make the studies work."

What kind of prayer works best? Colloquial and/or meditative prayer for guidance, a "Thy will be done" approach, appears to be more effective than ritualized or petitionary prayer in which a specific outcome is requested. Dr. Dossey, citing experiments done with a random event generator by Helmut Schmidt and Robert

Jahn's group at Princeton University, hints at mind-boggling possibilities that prayer can give us access to influencing events in the future and the past as well as in the present.

Regular practice of meditation can bestow health benefits similar to those demonstrated to result from prayer and an active religious or spiritual life. On CBS News with Dan Rather on January 15, 1996, Dr. William Shephard of the West Oakland Health Center in Oakland, California, presented documentation of a meditative technique that has been successful in significantly reducing hypertension in his patients. Dr. Dean Ornish's comprehensive program for reducing and reversing heart disease includes the practice of meditation. At the Menninger Foundation, meditation is used to improve immune function in patients suffering from AIDS, cancer, autoimmune diseases, and addictions, as well as for stress and anxiety. In a study conducted by Jon Kabat-Zinn, director of the Stress Reduction Clinic at the University of Massachusetts Medical Center, meditation helped reduce chronic pain.[89] Transcendental meditation, or TM, the most comprehensively studied of meditative techniques, has been shown in more than five hundred scientific studies conducted in thirty-three different countries, the results of which have been published in over one hundred journals, to have physiological and psychological benefits, including decreased stress, anxiety, and depression, in subjects from all cultural and ethnic groups.

Experiments have shown that when a subject enters a meditative state, the EEG wave patterns of the right and left hemispheres of the brain, which during ordinary waking consciousness tend to be uncoordinated, will become synchronized. During deep meditation, right and left hemisphere will fall into a nearly identical pattern. Most fascinating of all, in deep meditation the brain waves of an entire group of people can become synchronized. Through the use of dancing, chanting, breathing, drumming, fasting, and other stimuli, many cultures have found their way into an altered state of individual or group consciousness for the purpose of experiencing a transcendent state of healing and connection.

Love appears to foster the same kind of brain wave synchronization that occurs during deep meditation. In a brain-wave monitoring experiment conducted at the National University of Mexico, a young couple who were deeply in love were also very much "in tune" with each other on a bioelectrical level, demonstrating synchronized EEG patterns throughout the study.[90]

Mothers, twins, and lovers have long been noted for their ability to experience interpersonal connectedness that transcends space and time. I have had many experiences of this "knowing" connection with family members and loved ones.

Mitakuye oyasin. "We are all related." Love is the frequency through which we can connect and communicate with spirit, with each other, and with all forms of life. While the future of humanity holds many challenges, it holds tremendous promise as well.

So take a deep breath, relax, and enjoy the next few chapters on safe, low-cost, Earth-friendly, natural remedies that can be used at home. You're in good company. Including the populations of Japan, China, and India, where natural healing traditions are dominant, an estimated 2 billion people are using Earth-based remedies worldwide. The use of natural remedies that are responsibly produced can promote sustainable practices of stewardship and deepen our bond with our planetary home. Heal yourself, heal the Earth. As Ralph Waldo Emerson aptly observed more than a hundred years ago, "We have not inherited this planet from our parents; we are borrowing it from our children."

Exercise

"Your breath is your best friend and companion," Richard Baker, Abbot of the San Francisco Zen Center, stated recently on Jerry Brown's Oakland, California, radio show *We the People*. "You weave body and mind together with intention, attention, and breath."

Observing your own breathing is one of the oldest and most effective meditative techniques. Practice mindfulness simply by being aware of your breath as it enters and leaves your body. See how long you can remain aware of your breath in a twenty-four-hour period.

Breathing is by its very nature a form of at-one-ment, as that which we perceive to be outside of ourselves is drawn into our bodies and integrated. What are you breathing in? What are you breathing out? Set judgment aside and merely observe the process. Breathe in; breathe out. Breathe in; breathe out. Your breathing is one of the core rhythms of your existence. Under what conditions do you breathe fully and deeply? Under what conditions does your breath grow shallow or stop?

CHAPTER TWO

HERBS
Our Green Relatives

*Thank you for the healing ceremonies
and sweet medicines produced by
our green relatives who grow.*

—Russell Means, "Lakota Morning Prayer"

lants. They are everywhere, all around us. Even in the most barren concrete jungle, a careful eye can discern living bits of green, poking up intrepidly between sidewalk cracks or rapidly colonizing a vacant lot after a rain. Our "green relatives," as Russell Means refers to them in his "Lakota Morning Prayer," have been dwellers on this planet millions of years before we have. Herbs are humanity's oldest form of medicine, having been used for healing purposes for tens of thousands of years.

While the origins of herbalism are lost in the mists of time, some of the most ancient evidence of the medicinal use of plants was found in 1953 by Ralph Solecki and a group of archaeologists in the "cave of Shanidar" in the Zagros Mountains of Iran. Mingled in the ancient dust of the cave, along with the bodies of nine Neanderthals, was pollen from at least twenty-eight different species of flowers. Archaeologists deduced not only that wreaths had been made from these flowers to honor the dead, but that the plants were chosen because they were commonly known to have healing effects. Many of the plants, including yarrow and hollyhock, are still used medicinally by herbalists today, some sixty thousand years later!

Herbal medical traditions were already well established by the time people began to make and keep records of which plants were used for what purpose. One of the earliest such efforts was made by the Chinese emperor Ch'ien Nung more than four thousand years ago. His *Pen Ts'ao* herbal contains references to more than three hundred healing plants. Ayurveda, the traditional medicine of India that incorporates the use of herbs and aromatic essences, has been, according to astronomical records in the ancient Vedic texts, in practice since before 4000 B.C. The Ebers Papyrus contains details of ancient Egyptian herbology. Greek and Roman texts drew heavily on these earlier traditions.

At present, plants still play an important role even in modern allopathic medicine. Of 119 plant-derived pharmaceutical medicines, three quarters are used for purposes similar to their traditional uses among aboriginal cultures. Twenty-five percent of all prescription drugs contain one or more active ingredients derived from plants. Morphine, for example, is derived from the opium poppy, which was used medicinally by the ancient Babylonians. Vincristine, an alkaloid isolated from the Madagascar periwinkle, is used to treat childhood leukemia, and has increased the survival rate of children afflicted with the disease from 20 percent to an impressive 80 percent. Its use was discovered by a researcher working in a tiny plant medicine research department of a major pharmaceutical company. As one of the researchers himself described it, the budget for his department was so small it was listed in company reports under the category "miscellaneous."

A wide variety of herbal preparations are currently available in health food stores and alternative pharmacies. However, you are unlikely to find anyone working in the store or pharmacy who has any real training in the use and effects of all the herbs being sold there, and who would thus be qualified to advise you on the choice of herb and dosage. Some herbs do have side effects, though not generally of the intensity or seriousness of those caused by pharmaceutical drugs. Certain herbs can also change the way prescription or over-the-counter drugs are absorbed and used by the body. For example, goldenseal can alter the liver's metabolism of drugs, and cayenne and ephedra can alter gastrointestinal tract absorption. Some herbs are considered "plant drugs" and as such should not be used without professional guidance. It is best to consult with a trained herbalist or medical practitioner before adding herbs to your healing regimen.

WHEN TO USE HERBS

Most illnesses are self-limiting, and thus will go away all by themselves eventually. Natural healing attempts to shorten the duration of the illness, ease the symptoms, and restore balance to the system so that the body's natural healing ability is maximized. While illness is commonplace, it is not inevitable. An acute illness serves as a friendly reminder to us that something in our lives is out of balance and needs to be addressed. If we continue to ignore the problem, we can develop a chronic condition or a life-threatening disease.

According to Michael Moore of the Southwest College of Botanical Medicine in New Mexico, "Herbs work best on acute self-limiting problems and sub-acute or sub-clinical disease," or to put it even more simply, when we are "sick . . . but not *very* sick." For home use of herbs, this is a good rule of thumb. While natural healing methods can be quite successful in treating chronic or life-threatening disease, such situations are beyond the scope of this book and beyond the knowledge and ability of most laypeople to diagnose or treat at home. Part of being an effective home healer is being able to recognize when you're out of your league. If an illness persists or symptoms worsen, never hesitate to consult with a qualified medical practitioner.

That said, there are many symptoms that can be eased and conditions that can be treated at home with simple herbal teas, infusions, and tinctures that you can make yourself. Some herbs are best used fresh, such as lemon balm, which loses most of its delightful lemony scent in the process of desiccation, or lobelia, which loses its potency in drying. Conversely, there are other herbs that are best used when dried. Some herbs can be used either way.

A FEW WORDS ON WILDCRAFTING

Spending a day picking wild herbs in the open countryside is a healing adventure in and of itself. But make sure you know what you're doing! Never harvest a wild herb without being 100 percent certain of what you're taking. A number of commonly used herbs are now endangered as a result of overharvesting. Goldenseal is a prime example. Despite its usefulness and popularity, especially in tincture form combined with echinacea, I cannot recommend the use of goldenseal until such time as it is widely cultivated or it can be proven that the source from which it is derived is both legal and sustainable (much of the goldenseal on the market now is reputedly poached from northeastern forests). Other healing plants, such as the beautiful ladyslipper orchid, which grows wild in the woods of my native Wisconsin, are protected, and for good reason. Let such plants be.

Never take the only plant, or one of very few plants in an area, and never take anything from the "grandmother" or "grand-father" plant, the one that is obviously the strongest and best established, or "leader," of a group of similar plants. In many American Indian traditions, the "leader" plant would be given an offering of cornmeal or tobacco while a request was being made to harvest another plant within its "jurisdiction." As Wooden Leg, a nineteenth-century Cheyenne, described it, "The old Indian teaching was that it is wrong to tear loose from its place on the earth anything that may be growing there. It may be cut off, but it should not be uprooted. The trees and the grass have spirits. Whatever one of such growths may be destroyed by some good Indian, his act is done in sadness and with a prayer for forgive-ness because of his necessities."

If you are gathering in the countryside, or away from your own neighborhood, find out who the owner of the property is and ask permission before wildcrafting, even if it appears that no one "owns" the land. All the land in this country is either privately or government owned. If government owned, such as a state or national park, there is a good chance it is not legal to pick the plants. If privately owned, the identity of the owner can usually be discovered by asking the nearest neighbors. If the land is posted, do not trespass.

The energy of a wild plant is very different from that of a cultivated herb, which is not to say that it is always superior, just different. Examples of herbs that you may want to wildcraft, depending on where you live, include plentiful and useful plants such as fennel, miner's lettuce, mullein, mustard, wild mints, nettles, plantain, wild roses, mountain sage, or wild strawberries. Gather herbs away from heavily traveled areas, such as roadways used by cars and trucks or often-used footpaths that may be frequented by pet owners. Bring a notebook to record where you found the plant, its habitat and neighbors, the date and time, weather conditions, and anything else of significance.

Growing Your Own

It is impossible to describe to one who does not feel by instinct
"the lure of green things growing," the curious stimulation,
the sense of intoxication, of delight, brought by working among
such green-growing, sweet-scented things.

—Alice Morse Earle, *Old Time Gardens*

There are several good reasons to grow your own herbs. First, you can be assured that the herb you have is the herb you need. If you buy herbs, be warned that mistakes can happen. For example, it is estimated that a portion of the skullcap being sold by herb companies is actually germander, a similar plant for which it is often mistaken. Second, when using herbs medicinally, purity is of the utmost importance. Because of price considerations, much of the herbal material commercially available in the United States is actually grown in other countries and imported. Many of these countries have lax environmental regulations compared to the United States. They may routinely spray their herbs with pesticides, such as organophosphates (derived from nerve gas) and DDT. In China, India, and other parts of Asia, sources of many commonly used herbs, human feces is often used to fertilize the fields, creating a genuine risk of *E. coli* contamination in the final herbal product (there have been actual cases of this in the United States). Imported herbs are subject to fumigation and irradiation when they enter this country, and many are routinely sprayed with antibiotics. To reduce bacteria counts, large suppliers often spray with ethylene oxide, a carcinogenic gas that is believed to alter the healing constituents of the herbs.

The third reason to grow and make your own herbal medicines is potency. Even if you are lucky enough to find a commercial company selling authentic herbal products grown in the United States under pesticide-free, sanitary conditions, there is no guarantee that the herbs were harvested at the proper time, that they were dried correctly, or that tinctures were properly made. In addition, heat and light from industrial, mass-market oriented processing and packaging can seriously erode quality. Herbal preparations you make yourself will be fresher and more potent than those you would find in a store.

Herbs are easy to grow in most climate zones of the United States, as long as you observe the basics, such as matching the amount of sunlight and water preferred by the plant to its spot in your garden. For instance, you would not expect moisture- and shade-loving peppermint to grow alongside lavender, which flourishes in dry soil with lots of hot sun. Many herbs make excellent companions to flowers and vegetables: garlic, for example, improves the scent of roses, and gardening folklore claims that chamomile will strengthen weak or sickly plants growing nearby. Rosemary, which flourishes as a perennial here in the Mediterranean climate of southern California, can also be grown in more northerly climate zones if planted in a pot and brought indoors during the colder months.

Most herbs are hardy and forgiving and can be enjoyed throughout the growing season in fresh beverages and salads as well as soups and other dishes. On a summer morning or afternoon, you can take your teapot right out to the garden and pinch off a bit here and there of what looks good to you. Cover with hot water, steep for a few minutes, add a bit of honey if you like, and enjoy! There are few activities in life more rewarding than savoring a fresh herbal tea or a salad grown and gathered with your own hands.

It is a feeling like no other to sit or stand quietly in the midst of your own healthy garden at midsummer. When we cultivate a garden, we glimpse what it means to sustain creation, knowing that without our love, our planning, our intention and attention, this small pocket of life would not exist. Gardening, like parenting, is the patient nurturing of the potential of other life-forms. If done with conscious awareness, it, too, can be a form of healing through renewed attunement with natural forces.

If you live in an apartment or do not have an outdoor space appropriate for planting a garden, you can plant in containers such as half-barrels or window boxes. Many herbs can be grown from seed. If you have a very short growing season or more cash than time, you can also purchase young plants and nurture them quickly to lush maturity. This is a rich, all-purpose potting blend for use in pots, half-barrels, or window boxes.

Soil Mix for Container Herbs

2 parts potting soil
1 part perlite
1 part peat moss
1 part aged manure or compost

Potted Herbs: Herbs that have a difficult time surviving winter in a colder climate can be planted in containers and brought indoors when the weather becomes inhospitable. Grow bay laurel, scented geranium, ginger, rosemary, or pineapple sage in 12-inch pots with the soil mixture above. These herbs should last for three or four years before they need replacing.

Herbal Tea Barrel: Try planting a half-barrel with catnip, lemon balm, marjoram, mint, sage, and thyme. Or try growing one big single perennial, such as lavender. If you drill 2-inch holes on the south-facing side of the barrel, you can tuck compact clusters of a few extra herbs such as thyme, marjoram, or parsley into the holes.

Medicinal Window Box: An 8-inch-deep, 2-foot-long window box made of cedar or redwood will hold about a dozen annuals, planted four inches apart, in two rows (perennials tend to grow too large for window boxes, although trailing rosemary and thyme are possibilities). Try German chamomile, calendula flowers, basil, and lemon thyme, or several varieties of sage (pineapple, purple, and white) and thyme can go well together too. Thyme keeps very well in the freezer, and a hot, fresh-tasting cup of fortifying thyme tea with honey is most welcome during the winter cold and flu season.

Family Medicinal Garden: A full spectrum, multipurpose blend of healing herbs to be used fresh or dried after being grown in a home garden might include the following: basil, bay, calendula, catnip, German chamomile, chili peppers, chives, comfrey, dill, echinacea, garlic, ginger, lavender, lemon balm, lemon verbena, marjoram, mint (one or several of the many varieties available), mullein, parsley, rosemary, sage, sweet cicely, tarragon, thyme, yarrow.

Drying Herbs

Herbs for drying are best harvested at the peak of their potency, just before flowering. Harvest them on a sunny day, after the morning dew has dried. Check for insects and remove any wilted or insect-gnawed leaves. Gather and tie the herbs in bunches, then hang them in a warm, dry room or cupboard out of full sunlight for about two weeks. A garage or attic can serve nicely, or even a room that doesn't have a south-facing window. Herbs can also be dried on screens (you can make your own by stretching window screen over a nailed-together wooden frame) or in a slow oven, at 80–100 degrees for about an hour. Roots are usually harvested in the spring or fall, when the energy of the plant is concentrated there. In the summertime, the plant's energy tends to be more concentrated aboveground in the foliage or flower.

To store herbs, strip the dried leaves away from the stems and pack them into tight-sealing glass jars. Tall herbs, such as yarrow or lavender stalks, store nicely in tall glass pasta jars, which are often available in dark glass. Herbs with small leaves, like thyme or rosemary, store well in screw-top or corked spice jars.

Herbs can also be preserved in oils or vinegars, or made into salves, capsules, or tinctures. However you preserve them, just be certain to mark the container clearly with the name of the herb, the source, and the date. Kept out of direct sunlight, herbal oils can last for up to one year, herbal vinegars as long as two years. Dried herbs will begin to lose their potency within six months to a year, depending on the type of herb and the storage method used. Fortunately, tinctures can last indefinitely.

Making a Tincture

Tinctures are basically solvent extractions of the active ingredients of herbs and can be made with fresh or dry plant material. To use the old European method, begin the process of making a tincture with the new moon. For a fresh tincture, chop up the fresh plant material, then add one part herb (by weight) to two parts ethanol (by volume). In other words, one ounce of fresh chopped herb, weighed on a kitchen scale, would be combined with two ounces of ethanol, measured in a measuring cup. (If you have trouble getting ethanol, also known as Everclear, which is 190-proof alcohol and illegal in some states, substitute the highest-proof vodka or brandy you can find.) Let the mixture steep for two weeks, until the moon is full. Then pour off the tincture, filtering through muslin or cheesecloth, or a coffee filter (preferably unbleached), and squeeze out the sediment.

To make a dry tincture, or "maceration," the proportion of herb to solvent will generally be one to five. The percentage of alcohol in the solvent may vary depending on the formula or materia medica from which you are working. For example, "50 percent alcohol" means 50 percent alcohol, 50 percent water. Proportions will usually run between 50 and 70 percent. Again, begin preparations at the new moon. Prepare the dry herb by grinding it to a coarse powder with a mortar and pestle. (A small coffee grinder can also work very well for this purpose. For dried roots or berries, soak in alcohol for a few days before tincturing.) Put the dry herb into a glass jar. Add five parts solvent (by volume) to one part herb (by weight). Mix well, then tightly close the jar. Shake the mixture for a few minutes, twice a day, for ten to fourteen days. Let the solids settle for a day. Then pour off the clear tincture, filter, and squeeze out the sediment. Store in dark glass bottles.

Blender Method: Combine the herbs and alcohol in blender, and puree to a mash consistency. Pour into a jar and shake several times a day for two weeks, and then strain, squeeze, and bottle.

Double Strength Method: After straining out the original herbal material, add a fresh batch of herbs and let the mixture steep until the next full moon, filter, squeeze, and bottle.

Tinctures, when used medicinally, are generally administered in doses of 10 to 60 drops, or 1 to 3 droppersful, in a small glass of water or juice, every few hours.

To remove the alcohol content from the tincture, put the desired amount of tincture into a cup, then fill with hot water. The alcohol will evaporate. Drink what is left.

STANDARD INFUSION

This is the method for infusing most herbal flowers and leaves, such as chamomile, elder flowers, mint, rosemary, or cornsilk. Infusions can be drunk hot or cold as tea, or used for bathing, rinsing, or soaking affected parts.

Boil 1 quart water (32 parts by volume). Pour it over 1 ounce herb (one part by weight). Allow to steep for twenty to thirty minutes, then strain. Infusions should be made fresh daily, and the unused portion should be kept in the refrigerator.

DECOCTION

This method is generally used for roots, such as dandelion, echinacea, ginger, sarsaparilla, and sassafras. To 1 quart of water (32 parts by volume) add 1 ounce of herb (1 part by weight) and bring to a boil. Allow to boil for ten minutes, then turn off the flame and allow to cool. When cooled to warm, strain and bottle. To make a weak decoction, use half as much herb.

SYRUP

Syrups are particularly well suited for administering herbs to ease bronchial conditions, coughs, and sore throats, especially in children. To 1 quart of water (32 parts by volume) add 2 ounces of herb (2 parts by weight) and reduce until there is only 1 pint of liquid left. While the liquid is still warm, stir in 2 ounces of honey. Glycerin can also be used with or without the honey, and it gives the syrup a soothing texture.

HERBS AND KIDS

Herbs are an excellent way of supplementing a child's diet, especially when he or she is old enough to start making food choices out of parental sight or control. Tinctures can be added to juice or squirted directly into the mouth. Small children will often take herbal powders more readily if the herbs are mixed with applesauce or mashed ripe bananas. Many children will enjoy a pot of hot herbal tea with honey, especially at bedtime or during cold or rainy weather. Syrups made with sugar, honey, or maple syrup also provide a sweeter, easier way to make the medicine go down.

Dosage is based on the size of an average adult. An average adult weighs about one hundred fifty pounds. A child's dose is based on a fraction of this: a thirty-pound child takes one-fifth of an adult dose, a fifty-pound child takes one-third, and so on.

Herbs that act hormonally, such as black cohosh, ginseng, and damiana, should not be given to children, nor should any stimulant or psychoactive herb, such as ephedra, datura, mugwort, or yohimbe.

MOTHER EARTH'S TOP TWELVE HEALING HERBS

Aloe Vera *Aloe barbadensis*
The fresh gel is used as a poultice for chapped skin, dermatitis, eczema, and burns. The sap can be squeezed onto the area, or a whole leaf can be cut open, placed against the affected area, and bandaged into place. Aloe vera grows well indoors, or outdoors in frost-free climates. Mix aloe vera gel with glycerin for an effective moisturizer. **Sunburn gel:** I have used this many times to prevent peeling and skin damage from too much sun. The sooner it is used after the burn, the more effective it is. Scrape the pulp from a *fresh*-cut leaf of aloe vera and mix with one tablespoon of sweet almond (or other nourishing nut) oil and 10 drops of lavender essential oil. Spread liberally over sunburned skin and allow to soak in. Repeat application several hours later if possible.

Calendula (Marigold) *Calendula officinalis*
This beautiful, versatile healing flower has been used cosmetically, medicinally, and for cooking, as well as for decoration since ancient Egyptian times. Its leaves were used in the United States during the Civil War to treat open wounds. The petals can be used in cooking rice, cakes, breads, cheese or yogurt, fish or venison, and can be tossed fresh in salads. Steeped in an infusion, the flowers aid digestion and liver function and can be used as a rinse to brighten fair hair. Extract the oil from the petals by maceration in oil, and use for skin care, to soothe inflammations, chilblains, chapped lips, sore nipples (from breast-feeding), and diaper rash.

Cayenne *Capsicum annuum*
The botanical name for cayenne, or red pepper, is *capsicum,* derived from the Greek word for "bite." The potency of peppers is measured in heat units called "Scoville units," rating on a scale from zero (paprika) to three hundred thousand (Mexican habanero). Any red pepper with a heat rating of twenty-five or greater can be called cayenne. A member of the tomato family, cayenne is a favorite target of insects, so the crops tend to be

heavily sprayed, which is a good reason to try your hand at growing your own. Capsaicin, which gives peppers their heat, is an active ingredient of cayenne, and it has been shown to protect the DNA and cells from attack by toxic molecules such as environmental pollutants. By increasing blood flow and thereby improving the delivery of nutrients and the removal of waste from all areas of the body, cayenne has a positive effect on many conditions. Sprinkle powdered cayenne as a seasoning on food, or use fresh peppers in salads, hot sauce, and broths. String fresh peppers on cotton thread to dry, then pulverize and make into capsules. Cayenne is used as a folk medicine in Russia, where it is steeped in vodka and drunk by the glass. Fresh chili peppers contain more vitamin A and C than dried peppers. Cayenne is a carminative and stomach stimulant, promotes healthy digestion, and has been used for poor circulation, wounds, sinusitis, allergies, and to normalize blood pressure and cholesterol levels. **Caution:** Cayenne is best used in the short term for acute conditions. Excessive use may cause digestive, liver, or kidney disorders. Do not use if you suffer from ulcers. **Cayenne tincture:** Using a coffee grinder or mortar and pestle, powder dry cayenne peppers to a coarse consistency. Put 1 cup powdered dry cayenne peppers in a 1-quart glass jar. Add 1 cup 80-proof vodka. Blend fresh chilies with vodka in the blender to make 1 cup of mash and add to the contents of the glass jar. Top with vodka to make 1 quart. Shake daily for two weeks, strain, squeeze, and bottle.

Chamomile *Anthemis nobilis* (Roman), *Matricaria recutita,* or *M. chamomilla* (German)
Sweetly scented chamomile has been venerated throughout human history for its relaxing aroma and healing properties. It was the most valued medicinal herb of the ancient Egyptians and was used in Greece to treat fevers and female problems. Its name comes from the Greek *chamai,* meaning "on the ground," and *melon,* meaning "apple," indicative of the fruity aroma released when the plant is stepped on. Roman chamomile first appeared in England in the Middle Ages and, called "maythen," was one of nine sacred Anglo-Saxon herbs. This is also the chamomile that was trodden underfoot in lawns and gardens during Shakespeare's time. Historically, chamomile was smoked to relieve asthma. Known in gardening as a "physician" plant, it is believed to revive other weak or ailing plants near it. Roman chamomile tea is a

stomachic, treating dyspepsia and flatulence. German chamomile flowers are believed to make a better *tisane* (infusion). Large doses of either can cause nausea or vomiting. German chamomile is an annual plant, somewhat smaller than the perennial Roman. It grows wild in Asia, China, India, Australia, the United States, and Europe, where it is also widely cultivated.

Infuse the flowers to make a tonic, sedative tea that is especially effective for children and convalescents. As an eyebath, the infusion relieves inflammation and dark shadows. A chamomile compress aids in the healing of wounds and eczema. Use in the bath for sun- or wind-burned skin. **Chamomile eyebath:** First make an isotonic solution by mixing 1 teaspoon of salt in 1 quart of water. Heat this water to make an infusion with fresh or dried chamomile flowers. Strain through a coffee filter. Use as an eyewash for tired or inflamed eyes or mild conjunctivitis. Make a fresh infusion every five to six hours.

Echinacea *E. angustifolia, E. purpurea, E. pallida*
There are nine known species of echinacea, all native to the United States and used extensively by American Indians for a variety of healing purposes. *E. angustifolia* was favored by the Plains Indians, who used the plant for a variety of healing purposes, including wound healing and rattlesnake bites. The Choctaw used echinacea as a cough medicine and gastrointestinal aid, and the Dakota used it to treat diseases in their horses. At the turn of the century, echinacea tonic was the original "snake oil," popularized by a traveling salesman from Nebraska who let live rattlesnakes bite him during his sales pitch to demonstrate the efficacy of his tonic, the recipe for which was given to him by some Indian friends. After it purportedly cured the cancer of a prominent doctor's wife, echinacea tonic became extremely popular. Along with many forms of natural healing, echinacea was discredited by the American Medical Association (AMA) in the early 1900s, and the herb's healing properties were forgotten for many years. One of the best researched of immunostimulants, with over three hundred fifty scientific studies to back up its effectiveness, echinacea has been proven to boost immune system response by increasing T cell counts and macrophage production and activity, as well as boosting production of other immunity enhancers such as interferon and interleukin I. However, some research indicates that nonspecific immunostimulants, of which echinacea is one, cease

to stimulate immune response after a certain period, and therefore should not be taken for more than two weeks at a time. The most conservative research suggests the following dosage: three days on/three days off until symptoms improve. Echinacea can also be used externally for wounds, bites, and stings. It kills yeast and helps prevent infection by slowing or stopping the growth of bacteria and encouraging the growth of new tissue. To make a decoction, simmer five 1-inch pieces of root with 2 cups pure water for thirty minutes. Drink two or three times daily.

Garlic *Allium sativum*

Garlic has been in use as a medicinal for more than five thousand years. The healing properties of garlic have been used since Egyptian pyramid builders and Roman soldiers were given rations of garlic daily to fortify their health and ensure endurance. As a rule of thumb, the stronger it smells, the better it heals. (Eating parsley, chewing cardamom or fennel seeds, or using a tea tree or peppermint essential oil mouth freshener can help mask garlic breath.) Garlic is the most effective herb for killing bacteria, viruses, and fungi. A more potent antibiotic than penicillin, it destroys both gram-positive and gram-negative bacteria, including *streptococcus, staphylococcus,* typhoid, diphtheria, cholera, tuberculosis, and tetanus, among many others. Fresh garlic is a great antibacterial and viricidal. As little as 1 part in 125,000 will still have an antibacterial effect. Garlic is an effective blood cleanser, enhances immune response, and reduces blood pressure. Take as a preventative for the common cold, worms, and dysentery. (Three whole, raw garlic cloves a day, in a salad or as part of juiced vegetables, is considered a minimum therapeutic daily dose.) Plant garlic near roses to improve their scent, and under peach trees to avert leafcurl.

Ginger *Zingiber officinale*

Ginger is a perennial herb, first mentioned for its medicinal properties by Confucius half a millennium before the birth of Jesus. Arab traders brought it to the Mediterranean, and by the first century A.D. it was known to the Greeks and Romans as an aid to digestion. Its name is derived from the Sanskrit word *shringavera,* meaning "shaped like a deer's antlers," referring to the shape of the plant's root, or rhizome. Fresh ginger was touted as a medicinal that "eliminates body odor and puts a person in touch with the spiritual" in the *Pen Ts'ao* herbal of ancient China. It is currently cultivated throughout Asia, with half of the world's harvest coming from India. Jamaica is generally recognized as producing the finest ginger. Studies have confirmed what ancient Chinese sailors knew well regarding ginger's effectiveness in treating motion sickness. A standard dose for this purpose would be 1,000 to 1500 milligrams taken about half an hour before traveling. Taken in capsule form it may cause a mild burning sensation in people with sensitive stomachs. As an alternative to capsules, a cup of fresh ginger infusion will contain about two hundred fifty milligrams, while an eight-ounce glass of natural, authentic ginger ale will contain up to one thousand milligrams. Ginger can also be used to help relieve nausea caused by morning sickness or following anaesthesia. The herb has a beneficial effect on the stomach and gallbladder, stimulates digestion, and helps prevent ulcers. In nineteenth-century America, ginger powder or tea was used for infant diarrhea. Ginger's cardiotonic properties can help prevent angina and heart attack, as some of its active compounds slow and strengthen the heartbeat. It has also been used traditionally by the Chinese to ease menstrual cramps and arthritis. Fresh gingerroot that is juiced, infused, or decocted, is an excellent overall cleanser for the system. Its warming and immune-enhancing properties make it an excellent cold treatment. A bit of the root can be chewed to ease a sore throat. Dried or powdered ginger, rather than fresh, should be used to make a tea infusion for coughs. It can also be candied or used as a tincture.

Lavender *Lavandula angustifolia, L. officinalis, L. vera*
The Greeks and Romans used this herb extensively in bathing and washing, as reflected in its name, derived from the Latin *lavare,* meaning "to wash." The clean, refreshing smell of lavender has inspired its use as both a perfume and a medicinal. Fresh lavender was used as an infusion or flower water to bathe the temples during a headache or to cure lightheadedness. Dried stalks were placed among clothing and linen to repel insects such as moths and flies. An infusion of fresh or dried lavender flowers can be drunk as a tea to soothe headaches, calm nerves, and ease dizziness and flatulence. Lavender oil should not be taken internally unless prescribed. The herb also makes a sweet-smelling rinse for hair or clothing. Dried lavender flowers are a popular ingredient in potpourris, sleep pillows, and sachets. **Lavender Water:** You

can distill your own lavender water at home using an enameled teapot, a length of copper tubing, and a bowl of ice. Fill the teapot with fresh lavender, harvested as the purple flowers begin to open. Cover with water, and set on the flame to boil. Run a length of copper tubing (plastic tubing can get too hot and melt) from the spout of the teapot, down through the bowl of ice. Set the end of the pipe in a jug or bowl, and wait patiently for a couple of hours as the condensed distillate slowly drips out of the end of the pipe. A teapot full of lavender and water will yield about eight to twelve ounces of lavender water, and the house will smell wonderful while you're doing it. Flush out the copper tubing before using it again, to prevent metallic residue in the distillate.

Mint *Mentha* species
There are more than six hundred varieties of mint, leading a monk to declare over one thousand years ago that he would rather count the sparks of Vulcan's furnace than attempt to describe them all. Spearmint and peppermint, grown near roses, keep aphids away. Mint should be picked just before flowering, and it can be preserved by freezing, drying, or infusing. Macerated in oil, spearmint and peppermint make an excellent massage oil for migraines, neuralgia, and rheumatic or muscular aches. Spearmint is useful in a strong decoction to heal chapped hands or to refresh and reinvigorate in the bath. Peppermint speeds digestion and reduces acidity, making it an excellent remedy for holiday overindulgence. Cold peppermint tea reputedly gets rid of the hiccups. Pennyroyal is supposed to repel ants and fleas in the home. It should not be used during pregnancy, as both the American and European varieties have been used historically to promote menstruation. *Hederoma pulegoides,* or American Pennyroyal, was used by many native peoples as a children's remedy, for colic, headaches, measles, fevers, and restlessness. Pennyroyal oil should be used with caution. All mints are useful for their scent in potpourris and can be grown indoors.

Rosemary *Rosmarinus officinalis*
Native to the Mediterranean shores of France and Spain, rosemary first came to this country in 1606, and it has been cultivated here ever since, though it did not thrive in the harsh New England

winters of the early American colonies initially. Historically, rosemary has been used as a medicinal herb for more than two thousand years, and it was a popular feature of both weddings and funerals. Egyptians and Arabs grew rosemary in their gardens, Greeks used it as a disinfectant, and the Romans brought it to Britain, where it became a popular monastery medicinal herb during the Dark Ages. Rosemary has been used traditionally as a memory aid and refreshing herb, to uplift the spirits and to strengthen the heart. Branches of it were also burned in sick rooms, hospitals, jails, and courts of law to prevent the spread of "jail fever," or typhus. During the seventeenth century, it was used as a plague deterrent to be sniffed from the handles of walking sticks and small pouches. The fresh leaves, infused as a hot tea with honey, can be very soothing for colds, flu, and bronchial congestion, which I discovered accidentally when I sent a friend out to pick some of my fresh thyme to make me a tea when I was sick in bed. Not knowing herbs, he picked the rosemary by mistake (the plants grew next to each other) and dutifully made me a tea, which had a powerful reviving effect and noticeably relieved my bronchitis. (Again, do not take undiluted rosemary oil internally.) In the garden, rosemary companions well with sage. Rosemary was also a featured ingredient in "Hungary water," an early cologne. I have read several versions of the origin of this concoction, mostly described as a secret formula given to a thirteenth-century queen, Elizabeth of Hungary, by a hermit who assured her that it would preserve her beauty. Another version of the story claims the queen was paralyzed, and daily rubdowns with this recipe restored the use of her limbs. Whether for health or beauty, or both, here it is. **Hungary Water** (the queen's own formula, dated 1235): "1 gallon brandy or clean spirits, 1 handful of rosemary, 1 handful lavender, 1 handful myrtle. Handfuls are measured by cutting branches of herbs that are twelve inches long. A handful is the number of such branches that can be held in the hand. After measuring, the branches should be cut up into 1-inch pieces, and put to infuse in the brandy. You will then have the finest 'Hungary water' that can be made."

Sage *Salvia officinalis*
Another Mediterranean native, sage is a genus of the mint family and boasts more than five hundred species. The Latin name for sage is derived from *salveo,* meaning "to be well." John Hell, in

Virtues of British Herbs, describes fresh sage tea infused just as the flowers begin to open as a panacea: "one of the most delicious cordials that can be thought, warm and aromatic. Will retard the rapid progress of decay that treads the heels so fast in the latter years of life, will relieve that faintness, strengthen that weakness and prevent that sad depression of spirits, . . . will prevent the hands from trembling and the eyes from dimness and make the lamp of life, so long as nature lets it burn, burn brightly." Another medieval text puts it even more succinctly: "The desire of sage is to render man immortal." Sage has been used medicinally throughout Europe, China, and Persia. In this country, sage tea sweetened with maple sugar is a Vermont favorite. Sage tea after a meal helps digestion, and a tea or wine infusion functions as a blood and nerve tonic. Limit sage infusion to one week. Pregnant women should not use sage tea while nursing. Sage is also an antiseptic and antifungal and contains estrogen, which may be why Hippocrates insisted that women drink sage tea after wars, to get a head start on replenishing the thinned ranks.

Thyme *Thymus vulgaris*
In the first century A.D., Dioscorides prescribed thyme mixed with honey as a remedy for throat diseases and asthma. The Romans used thyme to banish melancholia, and in the thirteenth century Crescentius suggested, "If you drink the wine in which the herb is cooked, it will warm the heart, the liver, and the spleen." Roman soldiers bathed in thyme water to increase vigor and endurance, and the Greeks were fond of it as an ingredient in their after-bath massage oils. The Greek name for thyme is derived from a word meaning "to fumigate," attesting to its historical use as an antiseptic. Thyme is a good garden companion for lavender. **Guatemalan cough syrup:** Chop an onion, add to a saucepan of water, and bring to a boil. Simmer for twenty minutes, then add a handful of fresh thyme, or several tablespoons if dried. Let infuse for another ten minutes, then strain, add honey, and drink to alleviate cough.

OTHER USEFUL MEDICINAL HERBS FOR HOME USE

Anise *Pimpinella anisum*
Egyptians were cultivating anise for medicinal purposes as early as
1500 B.C. The herb was brought to America by the early colonists
and was a valued medicinal among the Shakers. Infuse the seeds
to make a tea to ease nausea, colds, coughs, and bronchitis, to
soothe colic in babies, and to increase milk supply in nursing
mothers. Can grow indoors. Do not confuse with Japanese Star
Anise, which is poisonous.

Astragalus *Astragalus membranaceus*
Used traditionally as a medicinal plant for thousands of years in
China and Asia, modern studies confirm that this root is a powerful and effective immunostimulant, increasing the number and
development of active immune cells, stimulating production of
interferon, and enhancing macrophage activity for up to three
days following its use.[1] It has also been found to inhibit the
growth of tumor cells in mice and to increase the life span of
human cells in culture.[2] A study at the University of Texas
Medical Center in Houston demonstrated that astragalus extract
was able to restore the function of damaged immune cells from
cancer patients, making them in some cases even more active than
immune cells from normal human subjects used as a control
group.[3] Chinese research shows that use of astragalus not only
reduces the number of common colds, but also shortens their
duration by almost half.[4]

Bay *Laurus nobilis*
Also known as "sweet bay" and "laurel," the bay tree was sacred to
Apollo, whose temple roof at Delphi was made entirely of bay
leaves. The oracle at Delphi consumed a bay leaf before going into
a prophetic trance, and a wreath of bay leaves, or "laurels," were
used to crown victorious athletes, soldiers, and poets as a symbol
of wisdom and glory, a meaning that is still preserved in scholarly
descriptions such as "baccalaureate." A decoction of bay leaves
can be added to the bath to relieve aches and pains. An infusion
can be taken to stimulate the appetite and aid digestion. The
leaves can be dried for use in cooking and can also be used to
flavor vinegar. Do not confuse Bay Laurel with Cherry or English
Laurel, which are poisonous.

Catnip *Nepeta cataria*
Dried leaves of catnip were once smoked as a mild hallucino-
genic. The fresh leaves contain vitamin C and can be infused to
relieve colds and fevers, to treat colic in children, and to be used
as a mild sedative. Used externally, the infusion can be massaged
into the head to relieve scalp irritations. Catnip repels rats and
can be planted near vegetables to keep away flea beetles. The catnip in my garden was always flattened down from the cat rubbing
his back into it. Looking for a gift for the cat who has everything?
Dry the leaves and stuff into homemade little pillows or toys.

Comfrey *Symphytum officinale*
Leaves and roots of comfrey contain allantoin, a component that
encourages healthy skin cell growth, which may be the source of
the plant's reputation as a healer. Popularly known as "boneset," it
was once used to help heal broken bones. An infusion of comfrey
leaf or root can be added to the bath to soften the skin. Fresh leaves
make an excellent poultice for aching joints, contusions, burns,
cuts, and sprains, and to reduce swelling. Internal use of comfrey is
not recommended, as the plant contains pyrrolizidine alkaloids,
long-term ingestion of which has been associated with chronic liver
and lung disease. According to the Henry Doubleday Research
Association, a group of comfrey growers and marketers in the
United Kingdom, "no human being or animal should eat, drink, or
take comfrey in any form" internally until further research has been
done on the cumulative chronic toxicity this herb may cause.

Dill *Anethum graveolens*
Dill was used as a soothing medicine by the ancient Egyptians.
Greeks used it to get rid of the hiccups. Do not plant near fennel
(they cross-pollinate). Seeds aid digestion, sweeten breath, and can be
infused as a nail bath to strengthen nails. Dill water (half an ounce
of bruised seeds infused in one cup boiling water, then strained) is
excellent for colic in babies, to increase milk flow in nursing
mothers, and generally soothes digestive problems and insomnia.

Elder *Sambucus nigra*
This perennial shrub was once associated with magic, the music
of flutes made from its branches being thought to attract spirits. It
was also used extensively for medicinal purposes and was known
as "the medicine chest of the country people." An infusion of the

dried flowers can be used to ease cold symptoms, especially when combined with peppermint and yarrow in a tea. The herbalist Roy Upton believes this to be a remedy superior to echinacea in the first stages of cold or flu and recommends drinking the hot tea while soaking in a bath of the same herbs to induce diaphoresis (sweating). Use an infusion of elder flowers and sassafras externally to treat acne. The berries are not good fresh, but are used dried and have a high vitamin C content. Blue elderberries are used in fruits and jams, though the red berries are poisonous. Elder leaves, roots, and bark should not be used internally. According to Indian tradition, elder is a women's tree, and only women should pick elder flowers, though men and boys are allowed to pick the berries. To use the flowers to ease female complaints, native tradition requires that the woman sing and pray while harvesting the flowers, having first left a tobacco offering for the ogimauikwe, or headwoman tree, which must be honored but not harvested from.

Elecampane   *Inula helenium*
This is another herb that has been used medicinally since ancient Rome. Candied elecampane root was sold in the Middle Ages to ease asthma and indigestion, particularly that caused by eating rich foods. A decoction of the root can be applied externally to acne or taken internally as an expectorant and digestive aid. Not to be grown indoors.

Fennel   *Foeniculum vulgare*
One of the oldest cultivated plants, fennel has been used traditionally since ancient Roman times to maintain good health and prevent obesity. Bruise the seeds and decoct to make an eye bath or anti-inflammatory compress. Chew seeds to sweeten breath and suppress appetite. Infuse seeds and drink as a tea to aid digestion and constipation.

Fenugreek   *Trigonella foenum-graecum*
Ancient Egyptians, Greeks, and Romans used fenugreek medicinally, though it is best known to modern herbalists as an herb that increases milk flow for nursing mothers. An infusion of the coarsely ground seed also stimulates digestion and eases flatulence and diarrhea. Mix crushed seeds with hot milk and apply to inflammations, swollen glands, sciatica, and bruises.

Ginseng *Eleutherococcus senticosus* (Siberian ginseng), *Panax ginseng* (Oriental ginseng), *P. quinquefolium* (American ginseng)
In China, where it has been used for thousands of years, ginseng is believed to restore balance and to increase strength and stamina by increasing yang energy in the body. The Soviet researcher I. Brekhman was the first to use the term "adaptogen" to describe the herb, meaning a substance that restores homeostasis and enhances endurance and resistance to stress. American ginseng was used by many native tribes of the southeastern United States, including the Cherokee, who considered it the chief of herbs and added a bit of it to most of their healing formulas. Ginseng became popular in America following the publication of an article by a Jesuit priest about its native uses. The root was decocted for colic in babies and drunk for asthma. An infusion of the leaf was used for coughs. The root was also chewed to ease nausea and vomiting, and applied fresh to sores.

Hops *Humulus lupulus*
A popular garden herb in ancient Rome, hops is best known today as a flavoring and preservative in beer. The flowers can be sprinkled with alcohol and combined with other soporific herbs in a sleeping pillow, or infused as a mild sedative and digestive aid.

Horehound *Marrubium vulgare*
Horehound has been used as a cough remedy since ancient Egyptian times. Its medicinal properties were known and respected by Hippocrates. An infusion of horehound, drunk cold, eases heartburn and is used to dispel intestinal worms. Horehound cough drops: Bring 2½ cups of pure water to a boil, while crushing ½ teaspoon of aniseed and 3 cardamom seeds in a mortar and pestle. Add crushed seeds to water, along with 3 ounces of freshly picked horehound leaves, 1 ounce of fresh thyme leaves, and 1 teaspoon grated lemon rind, and simmer below the boiling point for twenty minutes. Strain through cheesecloth or a coffee filter, then reheat the liquid and stir in 2 cups white sugar and 1½ cups brown sugar. Heat and thicken to the candy stage. Pour out onto an oiled cookie sheet and cut into cough-drop-sized pieces while still slightly warm.

Horseradish *Armoracia rusticana*
Roots can be stored whole in white wine vinegar or in sand. Chop

leaf and add to dog food to get rid of worms and improve muscle tone. Grated root makes a good poultice for chilblains, stiff muscles, sciatica, and rheumatism. It can also be eaten to stimulate digestion and eliminate mucus and waste fluids. Use in syrup for bronchitis and coughs. Do not grow indoors.

Kava kava *Piper methysticum*
As in North America, the island cultures of the Pacific region did not have any form of alcoholic beverage prior to contact with the Europeans in the eighteenth century. Imbibed socially by the ruling class, an infusion made from kava root was used in much the same way that wine was by the Europeans: to honor deities, visitors, and guests, to foster a warm social atmosphere, and to celebrate life events. Kava is also used traditionally for numerous medicinal purposes, including relaxation and weight loss. A 1996 double-blind, placebo-controlled study reported in the journal *Phytomedicine* confirmed the efficacy of kava extract in alleviating tension and anxiety. Speaking from personal experience, I find kava extract a wonderful stress-reliever with no mind-clouding or dulling side effects, although its use is not recommended for children or pregnant or lactating women.

Lemon Balm *Melissa officinalis*
According to Paracelsus, lemon balm is "the elixir of life," and when used as a morning tea with honey has been credited with bestowing youthfulness and extreme longevity on those who drink it. The herb was sacred to the temple of Diana and was used medicinally by the Greeks. Best used fresh, the lemony aroma is at its finest just before the flowers open. Fresh leaves can be used on bites and sores, and an infusion relieves bronchial congestion, colds, headaches, tension, and mild depression. This is an excellent bedtime tea for children and promotes sound sleep and pleasant dreams. Can be grown indoors.

Lemon Verbena *Aloysia triphylla (Lippia citriodora)*
Its beautiful lemon scent makes lemon verbena very useful for fresh teas and potpourris. It can also be infused in melted wax for forty-five minutes to scent candles. The infusion is mildly sedative, soothes bronchial and nasal congestion, and eases nausea, stomach cramps, and flatulence. Also useful as a skin toner and freshener. Dried leaves can be used in an herbal sleep pillow. May be grown indoors.

Lovage *Levisticum officinale*
This flavorful celery-like plant can be added to soups or steamed as a vegetable. Steep fresh seeds in brandy and sweeten with sugar for a digestive-aid cordial. Infuse the seeds, leaves, or root as a diuretic tea or systemic flush that can be helpful for rheumatism. The leaves can be frozen, the seeds and roots dried. Not to be used during pregnancy or if there is a history of kidney problems. Does not grow well indoors.

Marjoram/Oregano *Origanum* species
The name of this herb comes from the Greek *oros ganos,* meaning "joy of the mountain." Marjoram was once used to crown bridal couples. It was placed on graves to soothe the spirits of those who died. Leaves can be frozen or dried, or macerated in oil or vinegar. Infusion of oregano can be added to a relaxing bath or used as a hair conditioner. A tea infusion of marjoram eases colds, headaches, nervous tension, and rheumatic pain. An oregano infusion, drunk warm as tea, is said to prevent seasickness. Can be grown indoors.

Marshmallow *Althaea officinalis*
Marshmallow tea soothes coughs, diarrhea, and insomnia. A poultice of marshmallow soothes inflammations. Persians use it to soothe teething in babies. Boil root, skim off by-product, and use as a gentle cleanser for skin problems such as psoriasis.

Milk Thistle *Silybum marianum*
Aids in the regeneration of liver cells damaged by toxins and diseases such as hepatitis. Improves liver function.

Mustard *Brassica* species
Mustard has been used medicinally since prehistoric times. The flowers and young leaves can be used in salads. The crushed seed can be mixed with water and used as a deodorant, or to induce vomiting. A poultice of the powdered seeds can be used to relieve congestion in the lungs, arthritis, rheumatism, and chilblains. In a foot bath, mustard warms, soothes, and deodorizes feet and helps to relieve colds. The plant grows wild in many places and can be cultivated or grown indoors.

Myrtle *Myrtus communis*
In ancient Rome, myrtle was planted around the temples of Venus and was used traditionally in bridal feasts and wedding celebrations. The berries can be decocted as a rinse for dark hair. The leaves can be infused, fresh or dry, and used externally as an antiseptic and astringent, or internally for psoriasis and sinusitis. Can be grown indoors.

Nettle *Urtica dioica*
Nettles grow wild in many parts of the United States and can be used fresh in spring and summer, or frozen after a minute of parboiling for winter use. Rich in minerals, nettles are an excellent herb to use for enriching the blood. An infusion of nettle leaves is a remedy for dandruff and enhances the natural color of the hair.

Parsley *Petroselinum crispum*
The Greeks used parsley medicinally, although the Romans are believed to have been first to use it as a food. A handful of fresh parsley leaves contains a day's minimum requirement of vitamin C and can be eaten to freshen the breath and promote healthy skin. Infuse to make a hair tonic, facial steam for freckles, or soothing eyebath. Decoct the root to strengthen kidney function and as a mild laxative and anti-inflammatory. Grows well indoors.

St. John's Wort *Hypericum perforatum*
The medicinal parts of St. John's Wort are the tops and flowers, which release a blood-colored oil on August 29th, believed by Christians to be the day on which St. John the Baptist was beheaded. Flowers can be steeped in olive oil and placed in the sun for two weeks, at which point the flowers are removed and replaced with fresh blossoms until the desired potency is achieved. St. John's Wort oil has traditionally been used to ease sciatic pain, old sores, and wounds. A decoction can be used as a mouthwash for bad breath and gum problems. A tea or infusion can be made with one to two cups of flowers to one cup of boiling water and drunk three times daily to help alleviate depression, low self-esteem, and insomnia. A tincture can also be taken, twenty to forty drops, two to five times per day. It may take up to two weeks to notice the uplifting effect.

Sweet Cicely *Myrrhis odorata*
The fresh leaves can be used in salad. Infuse the clean, peeled root in wine or brandy. Old herbals describe it as a "tonic" for girls aged fifteen to eighteen. A decoction of the root is said to strengthen the elderly.

Tarragon *Artemisia dracunculus*
The leaves are nutritious and can be infused to make an appetite-stimulating tea. Also popular as a flavoring for vinegar. Leaves can be frozen or infused in oil or vinegar. Can be grown indoors.

Valerian *Valeriana officinalis*
Its name is derived from the Latin *valere,* meaning "to be in health," and it has been used all over the world since ancient times as a medicinal. Valerian was also used after World War I and II to treat shell shock and nervous stress. The root acts as a depressant on the central nervous system. Infuse in boiling water and let sit overnight, then drink as a mild sedative. **Insomnia tea:** One part German chamomile, one part St. John's Wort, one part skullcap, one part passionflower, one-eighth part valerian. Mix thoroughly and infuse to make a hot, soothing bedtime beverage. (Do not boil valerian root.) While most people find valerian to be soothing, even soporific, a small percentage may experience nervous agitation from its use. Check with your physician before using valerian. In large doses, it can cause headaches, restlessness, or hallucinations.

Vervain *Verbena officinalis*
The ancient Egyptians believed that vervain sprang from the tears of Isis, and among the Greeks the plant was sacred to Venus. The plant was used medicinally in China and had magical connotations for the Romans, Druids, Persians and Anglo-Saxons. The leaves can be infused in isotonic water for use as an eye compress or bath, or infused with rosemary for use as a hair tonic. The dried leaves can be made into a poultice and applied to wounds. A whole plant infusion makes a sedative bedtime tea that also detoxifies and promotes healthy digestion. Can be grown indoors.

Yarrow *Achillea millefolium*
Plant yarrow among other medicinal plants to increase their healing properties, fragrance, and flavor. Yarrow receives its Latin

name from the Greek warrior Achilles, who was said to have used it to heal wounds among his troops during the Trojan War. Yarrow stalks were used by Druids to divine weather, and in China to foretell future. Dry the flowering stalk and leaves to preserve. Infuse fresh flowers as a steam, toner, or pack for oily skin. Fresh leaves are hemostatic and can be pressed into small scrapes or cuts to stop bleeding. Yarrow tea helps digestion, alleviates abdominal bloating and gas, regulates menstrual flow, and helps break a fever and get rid of a cold. Among Native Americans, the leaves were chewed to relieve toothache, and the root was used as a mild local anesthetic. An infusion of the plant can also be used as a mouthwash for bleeding or inflamed gums. Among the Paiute, a strong yarrow tea was given to new mothers. Cannot be grown indoors.

HERBS TO AVOID DURING PREGNANCY

Aconite, black and blue cohosh, blue flag, buckthorn, cascara sagrada, chaparral, chokecherry, comfrey, damiana, datura/-jimson weed, dong quai, gingko biloba, ginseng, goldenseal, hellebore, horehound, immortal, jaborandi, juniper, kava kava, lily of the valley, ma huang/ephedra, mandrake, milk thistle, mistletoe, mugwort, parsley, pennyroyal, periwinkle, Peruvian (cinchona) bark, peyote, rue, saffron, scarlet pimpernel, shepherd's purse, sweet flag, tansy, tobacco, uva ursi, wormwood, yellow jasmine, yohimbe.

CHAPTER THREE

HOMEOPATHY
Similia Similibus Curentur

*T*he word *homeopathy* was coined in 1796 by Dr. Samuel Hahnemann to describe a new approach to medicine. Taken from the Greek *homoios,* meaning "similar," and *pathos,* meaning "suffering," the core principle of homeopathy is summed up by a Latin phrase also coined by Hahnemann: *Similia similibus curentur,* Like can cure like.

In Hahnemann's time, popular medical practices included bloodletting, electric shock, purgatives, and doses of poisonous substances such as mercury and arsenic. Before the days of germ theory and the discoveries of Louis Pasteur, these treatments were intended to remove from the patient the "cause" of the disease, which was believed to be contained somewhere within the fluids or contents of the body. Hahnemann, however, reasoned that the cause of any particular disease was removed in time and could not exist simultaneously with the effect. He came to the realization that symptoms were not the disease itself, but merely the results of the body's attempt to correct a "derangement" of spiritual or vital force.

Hahnemann also observed that relief of symptoms brought about by some of medicine's harsher practices were for the most part temporary and often resulted in greater suffering and deeper disease, even hastening death in many cases. Once the personal physician to German royalty, Dr. Hahnemann came to believe he was doing more harm than good to his patients and decided to leave the practice of medicine.

After leaving medicine, the multitalented Dr. Hahnemann earned a living by translating medical and literary texts. He was fluent in eight languages, had a strong interest in mineralogy and botany, and was the author of a respected text on chemistry. While translating *A Treatise on Materia Medica* by William Cullen, a prominent Scottish physiologist of the time, Hahnemann was troubled by a claim the book contained which stated that the effectiveness of Peruvian bark, also known as cinchona, used to treat malaria, was due to its bitter, astringent quality. In exploring the properties of cinchona and its effects on the disease, he administered small doses of Peruvian bark to himself and noted that it produced symptoms that resembled malaria.

He went on to test numerous substances in a similar fashion. Rather than test on those who were already ill or on laboratory animals, he gave doses of particular substances to healthy human subjects and monitored the effects. This method, known as "proving," is the basis by which the uses for homeopathic remedies were discovered. The results of numerous provings supported Hahnemann's theory that a substance in overdose produced certain symptoms in a healthy person that would (when administered in minuscule doses) stimulate the body's healing force in a sick person suffering from similar symptoms and effect a cure of the disease. "By observation, reflection, and experience," Hahnemann noted in his *Organon of Medicine*, "I discovered that, contrary to the old allopathic method, the true, the proper, the best mode of treatment is contained in the maxim: *To cure mildly, rapidly, certainly, and permanently, choose, in every case of disease, a medicine which can itself produce an affection similar to that sought to be cured!*"

By setting himself in direct opposition to conventional medicine, Hahnemann made a number of enemies for his new medical philosophy among those practicing the allopathy of the day. Homeopathy was flourishing in the United States after being brought here in the 1830s by Constantine Hering, a German immigrant. In 1844, Dr. Hering founded the American Institute of Homeopathy. The American Medical Association was formed three years later by conventional allopathic doctors, funded by drug companies. By 1900, homeopathy was more popular in America than in any other country of the world. Homeopathic medical schools sprang up all over the United States, training practitioners for more than one hundred homeopathic hospitals and more than a thousand homeopathic pharmacies. Fifteen percent of all American doctors were homeopaths. Then, early in this century, the AMA became a dedicated opponent of homeopathy and, in concert with several drug companies, engaged in a prolonged effort to discredit homeopaths and their practices. This, combined with the rise in drug-oriented medical treatment and antibiotics after World War II, resulted in the number of American homeopaths dwindling to less than two hundred by the 1950s.

Today homeopathy is experiencing a phenomenal growth in popularity once again. People all over the planet are currently receiving homeopathic treatment, the total number estimated at over 400 million. India boasts more than one hundred thousand homeopathic doctors and over one hundred four- to five-year homeopathic medical colleges. Mother Teresa offered homeopathic remedies at her missions. In Belgium, one person in four goes to a natural therapist, and homeopathy is the most popular treatment of choice. In France, where only 6 percent of the population had tried homeopathy in 1982, the number has increased to almost 40 percent according to recent surveys. There are now thousands of medical doctors and lay practitioners prescribing homeopathic remedies in the United States. Between 1980 and 1982, the number of American physicians specializing in homeopathy doubled. Sales of homeopathic remedies in the United States grew by 1,000 percent from the late 1970s to the early 1980s, with retail sales growing to $165 million in 1994. Other areas in which homeopathy is becoming increasingly popular are the United Kingdom, South Africa, Australia, Denmark, and the Netherlands.

Of the more than three thousand homeopathic remedies currently available, over 60 percent are derived from plants. Homeopathics are commonly available in the form of tiny pellets made of milk sugar that dissolve easily under the tongue. They can also be taken as tinctures, granules, or topical ointments.

Preparation of a homeopathic remedy involves a combination of dilution and vigorous shaking, called "sucussing." These two processes together form the basis of potentization, Hahnemann's method for diluting medicinal substances to prevent toxic symptoms while retaining their healing action. The more a remedy is potentized, the deeper and longer its healing action and the fewer the doses that need to be administered.

Substances used to create homeopathic remedies are diluted

in water or milk sugar. One part medicine to nine parts dilution are called decimal, or "x," potencies. One part substance to ninety-nine parts dilution are called centesimal, or "c," potencies. The fewer dilutions that have been performed, the lower the potency of the remedy. "X," or less than 30c, is considered a low potency. Dilutions to the thousandth part, the "m" dilutions, are considered the deepest acting and most therapeutic, generally to be prescribed by a homeopathic doctor or practitioner. For home use, homeopaths suggest potencies of 6x to 30c.

HOMEOPATHIC PRINCIPLES

Several concepts are integral to understanding the use of homeo-pathic remedies. According to homeopathic principles, people are considered "curable" if their constitution is "dynamic," defined as possessing the power of immune response, the power to resist disease. For such people, homeopathic remedies are effective in supporting the body's natural efforts by stimulating the existing resistance to disease. Those whose resistance is seriously impaired as a result of chronic disease or infection, or whose systems have been poisoned by environmental contaminants resulting in immune dysfunction, are said to have an "adynamic" constitution. An adynamic constitution will fail to respond to homeopathic remedies because there is little or no resistance left to stimulate.

Hahnemann defined a "cure" as "a recovery undisturbed by after-suffering." It may take more than one homeopathic remedy in the course of treatment to effect a genuine cure, as symptoms change in character. Dr. Hering, who brought homeopathy to the United States, formulated three guiding principles in the healing process that are known as Hering's Laws of Cure, based on his own observation and experiences as well as those of other physi-cians and practitioners.

The first of Hering's Laws states that healing begins in the deepest reaches of a person's being, the mental or emotional state and the vital organs, and moves outward to the more superficial or exterior parts, the skin, arms and hands, feet and legs. For example, an improvement in state of mind and overall outlook, such as the lifting of depression, accompanied by briefly worsen-ing symptoms in the physical body, such as aches and pains or a rash, would be considered an indication that a remedy is working. Hering's second law describes how symptoms often appear and disappear in reverse chronological order, as if working their way backward through time. The third principle states that healing usually progresses from the upper to the lower parts of the body, for example, a headache goes away, but arthritic-type pains are felt in the hands.

THE PLACEBO EFFECT

Does homeopathy really do anything? Or is its success simply a result of belief on the part of the overly credulous—the well-known placebo response? How does a homeopathic remedy have any actual effect on the human body when not a single molecule of the original substance from which it was made can be demonstrated to still exist within it?

Biophysics, a field of study that came into existence only within the last few decades, is believed to hold the answer to how vibratory therapies and energy medicine such as homeopathy, acupuncture, radionics, flower essences, and other subtle forms of healing may work. In the case of homeopathic remedies, the vibratory energy of the source substance is thought to imprint itself on the water molecules during succussion, when the molecules collide. This would explain why the higher homeopathic potencies, which have been succussed more, act more strongly and deeply, a fact that is borne out both by experience and by clinical research. Even though the highest-potency remedies are so diluted that they contain no physical trace of the original medicinal substance, the succussions have deeply embedded the energetic or vibratory imprint of the source substance into the diluent, thus increasing the remedy's healing power.

In an article published in the *British Medical Journal* in 1991, 107 clinical trials of homeopathy were reviewed: 77 percent indicated positive results for conditions ranging from asthma and flu to trauma, headache, and arthritis. Following are a few specific examples of some studies.

A randomized, double-blind, placebo-controlled study published in the *Lancet* in 1986 showed homeopathic treatment to be effective in lessening hay fever symptoms in 144 patients, following a brief initial aggravation of symptoms. The study concluded that placebo action could not fully explain the clinical response.

Another 1986 study published in *Psychopharmacology* showed that higher potencies of homeopathic remedies administered to white rats could be demonstrated to have a longer duration of effect than a lower potency.

A 1988 study conducted at the University of Paris and published in the *British Journal of Clinical Pharmacology* showed the remedy *Apis mellifica* to be an effective treatment for allergies. Apis mel. was also shown to be effective in reducing inflammation in a guinea pig in a 1989 French experiment. A double-blind, placebo-controlled 1990 study of the effect of aconite on reducing postoperative agitation in children yielded 95 percent positive results.

These are only a few examples of research confirming homeopathy's effectiveness. The more rigorously scientific, the higher the standards and quality of the methods in the studies conducted, the more likely homeopathic remedies are to show positive effects. As Hahnemann stated in his *Materia Medica Pura,* "This doctrine appeals solely to the verdict of experience. Repeat the experiments, it cries aloud, repeat them carefully and accurately, and you will find the doctrine confirmed at every step; and it does what no medical doctrine, no system of physic, no so-called therapeutics ever did or could do—it insists upon being judged by results."

WHEN AND HOW TO USE HOMEOPATHIC REMEDIES

Home use of homeopathics is best directed toward acute conditions and common ailments. Chronic ailments and diseases generally require constitutional treatment under the guidance of a trained homeopath.

The most important process in figuring out which homeopathic remedy to use is to create a complete listing of mental, emotional, and physical symptoms. A homeopath does this during a lengthy interview with the patient. Because we know the members of our own family so well and can readily observe them and any changes in their usual behavior, case-taking is somewhat simplified. Observe changes in appearance, whether the face is flushed or the pupils are dilated. Note any discharges, changes in sleeping patterns, whether symptoms worsen or improve in the morning or evening, or with exposure to heat or cold, or being indoors or in the open air. Is there irritability or sluggishness? Changes in mood or ability to concentrate? Are there unusual cravings for certain types of food, or hot or cold drinks?

When you have a complete list of symptoms, check through the remedy descriptions until you find one that matches all or most of what you have observed. (The listings of major symptoms and associated homeopathic remedies at the end of this chapter are for illustrative purposes. Complete listings of symptoms and applications for the remedies can be found in a good homeopathic materia medica accompanied by a repertory of symptoms.) There may be more symptoms indicated in the description of the remedy than you have on your list. You want to find the remedy that matches the most pronounced and important symptoms. In homeopathy, mental symptoms are considered the most serious, followed by emotional and then physical symptoms.

Use only one remedy at a time. For acute conditions, try a low potency (6x to 30c) of your chosen remedy every fifteen minutes to one hour. Start with one or two doses. If there is no change at all after six doses, discontinue the remedy and try another one. Stop administering the remedy when symptoms improve. If after you have stopped, the symptoms return, repeat the remedy using a higher potency. (Do not follow up with a lower potency.) In severe cases such as shock or trauma, use a high potency, such as 200x, administered once, possibly twice.

Homeopathics are excellent natural remedies for home use in the relief of common ailments. Because the cure is actually being effected by stimulating a person's natural resistance, the action of the remedies is comparatively gentle and noninvasive. Homeopathic remedies do not cause iatrogenic, or secondary diseases to develop. There are no serious side effects, although sometimes in the healing process there may be an initial aggravation of symptoms or, in accordance with Hering's Laws, a return of old symptoms in reverse order of their original appearance as the body works its way back to a state of healthy balance.

Homeopathics can be used with infants and the elderly and are easy to administer to children in the form of sweet pellets. The remedies are also useful for treating viral illnesses, such as colds and flu, for which there is no allopathic treatment, and for use in those who have allergies to allopathic drugs, such as antibiotics. Homeopathic remedies can also be used to support the body's natural healing functions during and after conventional medical treatment.

CARE OF HOMEOPATHIC REMEDIES

1. Keep remedies in a cool, dark place.
2. Do not store remedies near strong-smelling substances such as camphor, peppermint, clove, eucalyptus, menthol, moth balls, coffee, perfume, or incense.
3. Avoid handling remedies. Do not touch them with your hands. Pour the pellets into the cap of the container they came in, then tip them, untouched, into your mouth.
4. If a pill drops, throw it away.
5. When taking homeopathic remedies, avoid coffee (even decaf) or anything containing mint or eucalyptus, camphor, or cloves, such as candies, lip balms, muscle ointments, toothpaste, mouthwash, or tea. These substances may counter the beneficial effects of the remedies.

MOTHER EARTH'S TOP TWELVE HOMEOPATHIC REMEDIES

Aconite: This is a remedy to use at the very early stages of common illnesses such as colds or flu, at the first sign of fever, aches, or chills, or with a sudden drop in vitality, especially after dry, cold weather or exposure to drafts. Key indications are fear, anxiety, restlessness, sudden onset of symptoms, and thirst, sometimes intense, especially for cold drinks. There may be a sense of unreality and aversion to light, noises, music, touching, and smells due to oversensitivity. Anxious dreams are accompanied by tossing and turning. Also a good remedy following shock or disasters, such as earthquakes.

Physical Symptoms: Head feels hot and heavy, eyes may feel dry, gritty, and hot. Vomiting, perspiring. Rectal itching at night. Dry cough brought on by a chill, worse at night. Stiff, bruised feeling in the back and neck. Hot hands, cold feet, possibly tingling. Bad dreams. Fever alternating with chills, cold sweat. Dry mouth, white-coated tongue. Tingling, neuralgia. Dry, constricted throat. Colic not relieved by any change of position. With earache, outside of ear is red, hot, and inflamed.

Children: Watery diarrhea. Grabbing at the throat while coughing.

Worse: in a warm room and at night, especially after midnight, and from music, tobacco smoke, dry, cold wind.

Better: in the open air.

Apis Mellifica: Any condition resulting in symptoms that resemble a bee sting can benefit by apis.

Physical Symptoms: Swelling, edema, redness, soreness, stinging pain, aversion to heat and touch, with symptoms worsening in the afternoon. A person needing Apis may also be whiny, "childish," and apathetic, with a tendency to drop things. Sudden piercing screams, jealousy, and inability to concentrate are also mental symptoms. There may a craving for milk, but the person is not thirsty in general.

Worse: from heat, touch, after sleep.

Better: in cold air, after applications of cold.

Arnica: A first-aid remedy, for shock to the physical body, muscles and tissues in particular, following trauma, accidents, or surgery.

Physical Symptoms: Bruising, soreness, throbbing; the body feels as if it has been beaten. Also useful for those who are grieving or experiencing sudden financial loss, such as bankruptcy. Person may be unconscious or comatose but answers when spoken to. There may be agoraphobia and fear of being touched. A good remedy to take after childbirth, for after-pains or sore nipples.

Worse: from touch, movement, rest, after drinking wine, in damp cold.

Better: lying prostrate, with the head down lower than the feet.

Belladonna: Violence and the sudden onset of symptoms (always distinguished by hot, flushed skin, overexcitement, staring or glaring eyes, dry mouth accompanied by lack of thirst and no anxiety) are an indication of the need for this remedy.

Physical Symptoms: Upper lip may be swollen, pupils dilated. Painful earaches, with humming noises or pain that beats in time with the heart. Sore throat, worse on the right side. Tickling cough, worse at night. Glands may be swollen, extremities cold, though the skin is dry and hot. High fever without thirst, but feet are icy cold. May start while asleep.

Children: Very useful for type of fever and earache described. Also tantrums, biting, being lost in their own world, hallucinations of monsters. May be useful for teething.

Worse: from touch, noises, lying down, in the afternoon.

Better: sitting up in bed, warmth.

Symptoms needing Calcarea carbonica often manifest following treatment with belladonna.

Bryonia: Irritability and grumpiness, slowly developing symptoms and pains that get worse in the morning and with movement, are the hallmark of the need for Bryonia.

Physical Symptoms: Mucous membranes are dry, lips chapped. Stiffness in knees, at nape of neck, and in lower back. Splitting headache. Can be useful for breast engorgement in breast-feeding mothers and milk fever. Dry cough, worse at night, on entering a warm room or after eating or drinking, requiring counter-pressure on the sternum.

Children: Child is cranky and irritable and doesn't want to be picked up or carried.

Worse: from movement, heat or warmth, in the morning, after getting up or sitting up.

Better: pressure, rest, cold, lying on painful side.

Chamomilla: An especially useful remedy for children, but not for those who are gentle, calm, and mild-mannered by nature. This remedy is for crabby, irritable, whiny kids who are impatient, oversensitive, and snap or lash out at the slightest provocation. They tend to be complainers, do not want to listen, and especially hate being interrupted.

Physical Symptoms: In adults, a good remedy for coffee nerves. Colic accompanied by barking wall spiders (gaseous emissions). Earaches in which there is a feeling of heat and swelling, as if the ear is stopped up. Inability to tolerate pain (or anything else for that matter). Red cheeks, hot sweat, heavy perspiration at night. Sensitivity to smells. Headache on one side. Toothache that is worse after hot or warm drinks. Dry, tickling cough with tight chest. Inflamed nipples. Weakness in the ankles in the afternoon. Soles of the feet may feel very hot, especially at night. Disturbed sleep with scary dreams.

Children: Teething, tantrums, especially when the child wants to be picked up and carried everywhere. Calm children, especially those with a tendency toward constipation, do not need *Chamomilla.*

Worse: at night, in hot or windy weather, outside, when angry.

Better: in warm, wet weather, when carried or held.

Hypericum: Specific to injuries of the nerves, especially due to smashed fingers or toes, animal bites, and puncture wounds. An excellent first-aid remedy and companion to aconite in cases involving trauma and shock, such as after an accident.

Physical Symptoms: The head may feel elongated, with dull pain in the right side of the face. There may the illusion of being high up in the air or about to fall from a great height. Scalp may be sweaty, hair may fall out following injury. Also for nausea, hemorrhoids, herpes zoster, and asthma that gets worse in damp or foggy weather. Injuries to the base of the spine from a fall. Muscle spasms and twitching. Traveling pains. There may be thirst and a desire for wine. The tip of the tongue looks normal, but there is white coating toward the back.

Worse: from touch, in damp, cold, or foggy weather, in an enclosed space.

Better: from leaning the head backward.

Ignatia: This remedy is primarily indicated by moody, change-able, and erratic emotional states, especially those of sensitive, intelligent, excitable women whose natures are basically mild.

Physical Symptoms: The state of mind is introspective, sad, even to the point of tears, but with little desire to communicate. The attention is turned inward as a result of grief, shock, or extreme disappointment. They may sigh frequently. Sour burps, a feeling of emptiness in the stomach, hiccups, cramps, barking wall spiders. Much yawning, but sleep is superficial, and insomnia may be a problem. Tobacco smoke and coffee may cause headache that gets worse when bending over. There may be diarrhea and pain after bowel movements.

Worse: early in the day, outside, after eating, drinking, or smoking.

Better: while eating, warmth.

Nux Vomica: This is a commonly used remedy in homeopathy due to the many symptoms of common illnesses and modern living that it covers, and is especially indicated for males. A person benefiting from Nux vomica will generally be a white-collar worker or professional or businessperson who spends a lot of time indoors and leads a sedentary lifestyle in which the brain is used more than the body. Such a person is thin and active, with a tendency to be crabby. As a result of stress, he or she may try to regain balance or calm by indulging in alcohol, coffee, cigarettes, or drugs. Particular indications are crabbiness, oversensitivity to sound, smell, light, and touch, a sullen mood with critical remarks to the point of being mean or nasty. It can also be used for a hangover.

Physical Symptoms: Headache, especially when out in the sun, made worse by coughing. Sensitive scalp, dizziness. Colds in which a stuffed-up nose is worse at night or while outside. Itching or tickling in the throat after getting up in the morning. Nausea or vomiting after eating. Sore feeling in the midsection. Hangover that includes diarrhea. Itching hemorrhoids. May wake up at 3 A.M., get back to sleep, and wake later feeling terrible. Face and body may feel very hot, but taking off covers produces chills. Fingernails look blue.

Worse: in the morning, after thinking or studying, being touched, in cold or dry weather, after eating spicy food or taking drugs, coffee, or alcohol.

Better: after a nap, and in rainy weather, in the evening.

Pulsatilla: This remedy is indicated for sweet, gentle, emotional people, especially when they're feeling weepy. They very much enjoy receiving sympathy and comfort from others in this state. The person will feel much better when outside in the open air. She or he may be fearful and insecure, with a dread of the opposite sex. Pulsatilla types may also have a hard time standing up for themselves and a tendency to be bullied into going along with what others say, want, or do. They are changeable and may contradict themselves frequently. Symptoms are also changeable.

Physical Symptoms: Tension headache, styes, inflamed eyelids. Thick, yellowish discharges from eyes or nose, worse in the morning. Earache that gets worse at night, with a sensation that the ear canal is blocked, especially accompanying a cold. Outer ear is red and swollen, with a thick discharge that smells unpleasant. Mouth is dry, tongue coated white or yellow, lower lip may be swollen and cracked in the middle. Bad breath. No sense of taste, or food may taste different. Dislike of warm food or drinks, butter and fats. No thirst. Digestive problems, with rumbling in stomach. Several bowel movements daily. Dry cough in the evening, though thick, greenish expectoration may be coughed up in the morning. May feel sleepy in the afternoon, wide awake at night. Sleeps with arms raised above the head. Swelling in the knees and feet. Fever accompanied by chills in the late afternoon, feeling very hot at night.

Children: A craving for hugs and attention, fear of ghosts or of the dark.

Worse: from warmth, at night, from rich food, after eating.
Better: in the open air, while moving, from cool applications, food, or drink.

Rhus Tox: This remedy is particularly effective for joints and tendons, "rusty-type" rheumatic pains and stiffness that get better with stretching and movement. Also good for muscle strains as a result of heavy lifting. A person needing Rhus tox will have a hard time sitting still, always changing position to become more comfortable, tossing and turning and getting out of bed at night. There may be sadness and thoughts of "ending it all."
Physical Symptoms: Head feels heavy and as if brain is rattling, scalp sensitive, pain that moves from the forehead back. Colds caught from getting wet. Cellulite. Eyes may be swollen, red, sensitive to light. Earache with feeling that something is stuck in the ear canal, swelling in the earlobes, possible bloody discharge. Nose swollen and red, especially at the tip. Sore throat with swollen glands. No appetite, but heavy thirst, especially for milk. Bloated and sleepy after eating. Fever blisters. Diarrhea. Dry cough after midnight. Cold air causes pain and stiffness in arms and legs. Stiffness in the small of the back and nape of the neck, improved by lying on a hard surface. Cannot fall asleep until after midnight, then sleeps very deeply, with dreams of hard labor or taxing endeavors.
Worse: in or after rainy weather, while resting or sleeping on back or right side.
Better: in warm, fair weather, while moving, stretching, or rubbing, from warm applications.

Sulfur: Aversion to water or bathing, hot, burning skin, a tendency to take short naps, bright red lips, and a sinking feeling inside in the late morning all indicate a need for this remedy. A person needing sulfur will be lazy, self-centered, crabby, depressed, absent-minded, and weak. They may be "pig-pen" types and feel worst when having to stand up for any protracted period of time. Delusions, irritability, lack of consideration for others, and childish temperamentalism in adults are also indications. When ailments tend to recur, sulfur can be a good finishing remedy.
Physical Symptoms: There may be a hot or burning sensation on top of the head. Scalp is dry and itchy. Eyes burn. Extremely sensitive to smells. With a cold, there is oversensitivity to sound

followed by deafness. Lips are red and burning, tongue looks white, though the sides and tip are red. Gums may be swollen. Extreme thirst. No appetite, or ravenous hunger. Red, itchy anus. Feeling that something is sitting on the chest. Mucus rattles. May want window open to help breathing. Poor posture. Hot, sweaty hands. Very light sleep, may talk or twitch, intense dreaming. Insomnia between 2 and 5 A.M. Underarm perspiration smelling of garlic. Hot flashes. Dry, itching, burning skin that infects easily and gets worse from scratching and bathing.

Children: "Pig-pen" types, may be afraid to have bowel movements, good appetite.

Worse: in the morning, while standing, at 11 A.M., from alcohol, recurring.

Better: in warm, fair weather, while lying on the right side.

ADDITIONAL USEFUL HOMEOPATHIC REMEDIES

Allium cepa: Symptoms resemble what happens when you cut up onions: streaming tears and nasal mucus, burning discharge from nose, laryngitis, hayfever.

Alumina: Overall indication is dryness of mucous membranes, skin. The materia medica suggests this remedy for delicate children who may be suffering the ill effects of poor diet, especially those disposed to frequent head colds. Constipation in infants. Poor appetite, abnormal cravings, such as for chalk, charcoal, dry food, tea grounds. Potatoes make them feel worse. Debilitated elderly or prematurely old people who feel cold, depressed, and always in a hurry, though time seems to pass slowly for them.

Antimonium crudum: Most important symptoms are extreme crankiness and fretfulness with a thick white coating on the tongue. Whatever the condition, it will have these characteristics and will be made worse by heat and bathing. There may by canker sores and cracked skin at the corners of the mouth, inflamed eyelids, loss of appetite. Craving for acidic foods and pickles. Bloating or heartburn after eating and burps that taste of what was eaten. Diarrhea, especially after acid foods or baths, alternating with constipation. Headaches, especially after eating candy. Itching in chest. Sleepiness in old people. Pain in the fingers. Worse in the evening, better in open air and while resting.

Antimonium tartaricum: Similar to Antimonium crudum, with white-coated tongue, but distinguished by irresistible desire to sleep. Weakness, perspiration, and rattling mucus that cannot be loosened by coughing. In addition to desire for acid foods, there may be cravings for apples or fruits and cold water.

Arsenicum album: The hallmarks of need for this remedy are extreme weakness, exhaustion from any kind of effort, and restlessness, growing worse at night. Fearfulness, anguish, cold sweat, inability to stay still. There may be suicidal feelings and despair, along with a belief that medication is useless. Intense thirst but aversion to food. May crave milk and coffee. Vegetables, melons, vinegar, acids, and watery fruits cause stomach distress. Aversion to light. Puffy eyes and face, itchy, extremely sensitive scalp with dandruff. Also indicated for hallucinations, especially delirium tremens and other symptoms resulting from alcoholism. Disorder and confusion also make this kind of person worse. Symptoms are worse after midnight, in cold, wet weather, from cold drinks, near the ocean, and on the right side of the body. Better from heat, with the head up, and after warm drinks. Can be used to facilitate a peaceful transition to death.

Borax: Children needing Borax have a fear of being set down or carried downstairs, and will be very sensitive to sudden noises, such as thunder. A baby who cries when nursing due to thrush or soreness of the mouth may benefit from this remedy as well. Ends of hair may be tangled. Inability to sleep due to hot weather. Herpes, cold sores, psoriasis. For skin conditions, it can be used for several weeks.

Caladium seguinum: A smoker's remedy, to lessen tobacco cravings. Also useful for insect bites or rashes accompanied by intense burning or itching.

Calcarea carbonica: One of Hahnemann's original constitutional remedies. Overweight kids who eat too much junk food can benefit from this remedy, especially if they are fair skinned, sweat a lot, are easily winded, and prone to catching colds. They may crave eggs and eat dirt. Also useful for states of exhaustion caused by overwork, and for those who are fearful and absentminded, stubborn, and lazy. Pupils are dilated, eyelids itchy. A sour taste in the mouth, bleeding gums, and bad breath. Dislike of meat and fat. Thirsty for cold drinks. Night cough, aggravated by eating or playing piano. Sensitivity of chest. Cold feet. Easily startled. Overactive thinking makes it hard to fall asleep. Sleepy in early evening, but wakes often at night, with nightmares or dreams of people who have died. Swollen glands. Warts on face or hands. Worse from exercise and heavy thinking, cold, and during the full moon. Better in dry weather.

Calcarea phosphorica: Indications for this remedy are similar to Calcarea carbonica, but particularly indicated for teething, especially if the teeth are late in coming in, and for anemic children with digestive problems. A baby needing this remedy will want to nurse all the time, then spit up. Also for a child prone to throwing up. There may be desire for smoked or nitrite-heavy foods such as ham, bacon, or smoked fish. Stinky barking wall spiders (odorous flatulence).

Cantharis: Almost unbearable, constant feeling of the need to urinate, with pain before, during, and after, and scanty output of urine, sometimes only drops. Cutting, burning pains in the area of the kidneys. Heartburn and sour stomach during pregnancy. Sunburn and scalds. Worse from touch, urination, cold drinks. Better from rubbing.

Causticum: A child needing this remedy may have been a late walker. He or she may be afraid to sleep alone, wet the bed, feel sad, tearful, hopeless, and overly sympathetic toward others. Ringing or roaring in the ears, impacted ear wax. Runny nose, hoarse. Cough accompanied by pain in the left hip. Difficulty staying awake. May bite insides of cheeks. Dislikes sweets. Stiff feeling between shoulders, with pain at the nape of the neck. Useful for those who have worn out their voice, such as singers and speakers (try also a small piece of Borax). Suggested for dark-complexioned, thin (from worry, nervousness, or illness), taut people with sallow, pale, dirty-looking skin, possibly with facial warts. Symptoms worse from motion and in clear, dry, or windy weather. Better from warmth, in rainy weather, and in bed.

Cina: Described as a children's remedy, especially for infestation with worms and intestinal problems. The child needing this remedy is in an ugly mood and may feel or behave as if guilty of a crime. The child may want to be rocked but not otherwise touched or carried. May ask for one thing after another, rejecting them as soon as she or he has them. Intense nosepicking is characteristic, also itching of the anus and inside the ears. The abdomen may be tight and bloated, with pain around the belly button. Dark rings around the eyes, red cheeks. Coughing followed by gurgling down to the stomach. Fever in which face is cool, possibly with cold sweat, and hands are warm. Twitching, starting, and spastic movements, especially of right hand and left foot. Night terrors, talking, crying out, or gritting teeth while asleep. Sleeps on abdomen, may get up on hands and knees while sleeping. Worse at night, in the sun, in summer.

Coffea cruda: Nervousness, agitation, inability to tolerate pain, and overstimulation can indicate the need for this remedy. The mind is quick, happy, and full of ideas, making it difficult to sleep, especially after 3 A.M. Overexcitement and rapid heartbeat caused by joyful news or surprise. Headache that feels like a nail is being driven into the brain. Anal itching. Worse from strong smells, cold, open air, and at night. Better from warmth and lying down. Camphor and Cocculus should not be used with Coffea.

Colocynthis: Intense abdominal pain that causes the sufferer to double up is the characteristic symptom for this remedy. Useful for colic in infants. The person is very cranky, hates to be questioned. May feel dizzy when turning head toward the left. Bitter taste in the mouth. Pains in the calves of the legs may accompany colic. Worse on getting angry. Better with warmth, and pressure against the abdomen from doubling up.

Drosera: Hahnemann's primary remedy for whooping cough. The child may be dizzy when walking outdoors and fall to the left. The left half of the face may be cold while the right side is hot and dry. Worse from talking, singing, laughing, drinking, and lying down, and after midnight.

Euphrasia: Conjunctivitis, cold in the eye. There may be a bursting headache, with watery eyes and runny nose. Eyelids feel hot and swollen. Sleepy in the daytime, yawning when walking outside. Perspiration on the chest while sleeping at night. Worse from light, in the evening, from warmth, in the house. Better in the dark and after drinking coffee.

Gelsemium: Dizziness and trembling, muscular weakness, sunstroke, flu. Sickness that comes on after too much emotional excitement. Stage fright. The person needing this remedy will be listless, apathetic, quiet, and want to be left alone. Headache with pain in the temples and/or muscle tension in the shoulders and neck. Eyes may feel heavy. Tonsils swollen, with itching in the soft palate and sensation of a lump in the throat. Sore throat extending to the ear. Bad breath, bad taste in the mouth. Nervous diarrhea. Insomnia. Feelings of weakness and shakiness in arms or legs, with a desire to be held. Writer's cramp. Measles. Chills up the length of the spine. Worse from damp, foggy weather, before an electrical storm, from smoking, overexcitement, bad news, and at 10 A.M. Better in the open air.

Hepar sulphuris calcareum: Also known as "Hahnemann's Calcium Sulfide." Specific to unhealthy skin prone to infections. Indicated for impressionable, sedentary, blond-haired people. There is a tendency toward depression that is worse at night, with extreme irritability. Hay fever. Discharges that smell like old cheese. Chapped skin or lips, particularly a crack in the middle of the lower lip. Painful cold sores, possibly in the corners of the mouth. Loss of voice after exposure to cold, dry wind. Coughing to the point of choking when any part of the body is exposed to cold, or after eating cold food. Asthma that gets worse in dry, cold air. Fever with profuse sweating. Sour-smelling perspiration. Worse from touch, cold drafts, or wind. Better from warmth, covering the head, after eating warm foods, in humidity.

Ipecacuanha: Indicated for persistent nausea and vomiting, such as that caused by morning sickness or difficult to digest food. A person who needs this remedy may feel irritable and contemptuous. The eyes may be red, surrounded by blue rings, the face pale. The tongue will usually look clear, with abundant saliva in the mouth. Nausea gets worse during certain times of day, when lying down, or from damp, warm air.

Kali phosphoricum: An excellent remedy for extreme nervousness and depression brought on by overwork, overextending, excitement, or worry. A person needing Kali phosphoricum will be irritable, easily startled, have difficulty sleeping due to nightmares, and may feel that something awful is about to happen. There may be sleepwalking, loss of memory, and an aversion to being with or meeting people. Depression may be related to business problems. Any effort may seem to be too much. Bad breath, bleeding gums, foul-smelling excrement, yellow urine. There may be shortness of breath when climbing stairs. Temperature below normal. All symptoms worse from cold, in the early morning, and from exertion of any kind. Better with warmth and rest.

Ledum: This remedy is particular to puncture wounds or bites, such as spider bites, especially if the wounded parts feel cold. Nosebleeds. Dizziness, with a tendency to fall to one side while walking. Aching eyes. Acne on cheeks and forehead. Anal pain. There may be swelling in the big toe and ankles. Symptoms are worse at night and in a warm bed. Better from soaking feet in cool water.

Lycopodium: Symptoms requiring use of this remedy will tend to be on the right side of the body, and worse in the late afternoon and evening, from 4 P.M. to 8 P.M. Lycopodium types are very intelligent or precocious but physically undeveloped or weak, and thin to emaciated. They will not like being alone and distrust their own abilities. Small things bother them, and they prefer that with which they are familiar. Memory may be weak, with mistakes made in spelling and messy handwriting. They wake up sad and are afraid they will crack under pressure. Teeth may be overly sensitive. Tongue prone to canker sores. They prefer hot food and drinks, eat little and fill up fast, bloating after a meal, and may experience heartburn. Stools are hard and small. There may be night coughing with salty expectoration. Chills experienced between 3 P.M. and 4 P.M., followed by perspiration. They may be sleepy in the daytime and dream about accidents. One foot may be hot while the other is cold. Sweaty feet, dry palms, smelly perspiration. Symptoms are worse on the right side, between 4 P.M. and 8 P.M., from heat and in bed. Better from movement and after midnight.

Natrum muriaticum: This remedy excels at stopping a cold that begins with sneezing. Illness may be brought on by fright, grief, or an attack of anger. The person gets upset over nothing and wants to be left alone to cry. Tears may alternate with laughter. Eyes feel sore, especially when looking down. In children there may be a headache. Coughing causes eyes to water heavily. Heavy discharge of clear, thin mucus from the nose and a loss of the senses of smell and taste. Intense thirst and craving for salty foods. Dislike of bread, fats, wet, slimy foods. Chills may be felt between 9 A.M. and 11 A.M. accompanied by sleepiness. Hands may be hot and sweaty and the body is cold. Symptoms worse around 10 A.M., near the ocean, while talking, from heat, noise, or music. Better in the open air, after a cool bath, while lying on the right side.

Sabadilla: Specific for hay fever, especially when accompanied by nervousness. Also for sensitivity to cold, and diarrhea in children accompanied by cutting pains. There may be dizziness, sneezing, red, burning, watery eyes, clear discharge from the nose. Sore throat starts on the left side and feels better after warm food or drinks. Frequent swallowing. No thirst but wants hot drinks. Fever accompanied by chills, with hot head and cold hands and feet. Nails may be thick, while skin dry and cracked under the toes. Anal itching. Worse at the full moon and from anything cold. Better when bundled up, and after warm food or drinks.

CHAPTER FOUR

FLOWER ESSENCES

Nature Is Simple

No science, no knowledge is necessary,
apart from the simple methods described herein;
and they who will obtain the greatest benefit
from this God-sent Gift will be those who
keep it pure as it is; free from science, free from
theories, for everything in Nature is simple.

—Edward Bach, *The Twelve Healers and Other Remedies*

 hortly before I began to study flower essences, I had an interesting experience. It was springtime in Los Angeles, normally a cheerful time of year for me, a season of blooming flowers and green things growing, sandwiched between the wet southern California winter and the parched landscape of summer. Yet I was depressed, for no particular reason, with a sudden heaviness of mood that I endeavored in vain to talk and think away. Finally I felt that a walk in the fresh air might do me good. I headed for the nearest green haven, a small preserve in Coldwater Canyon owned by the Treepeople, a group dedicated to the planting of trees in the city.

Turning off the main trail to a smaller path that led up, I suddenly found myself on a hilltop, in the midst of a field of bright blooming plants that hugged the trail closely on either side, forming a kind of flowery tunnel. The plants were thriving, taller than I, graceful, upright stalks covered with tiny yellow flowers. As I moved delightedly through, butterflies flitted and bees buzzed. The view of the city in the valley below was totally obscured; nothing but flowers as far as my eye could see. It was magical. A childlike joyfulness blossomed in my heart. As the slender stalks brushed against me in the gentle breeze, it felt as if they were literally scrubbing away my dark mood. Silently I thanked them, dubbed the place "the Flower Forest," and vowed to bring my children there with me the next time. (They came, and spent the better part of the walk worrying aloud about whether or not they would be stung by a bee.) Later I learned that the yellow blooming plants of the Flower Forest were mustard, used in the Bach flower remedies for states of sudden, inexplicable gloom or despair.

What Is a Flower Essence?

A flower essence is water that has been impregnated with the vital force of a plant or tree, and preserved with alcohol, usually brandy. Flower essences differ from herbal tinctures or macerations in that only the flowers in perfect bloom, considered to represent the height of the plant's strength and potential for life, are used. The best of the flower heads are cut and floated on the surface of a clear glass bowl filled with pure spring water and left for several hours while the sun charges the water with the plant's particular energy. This, the "mother tincture," is then preserved with an equal amount of brandy and further diluted to create "stock" and "dosage" bottles. "Stock" bottles are the first dilution, and are generally kept by practitioners. "Dosage" bottles are a further dilution appropriate for administering as a treatment and are the form of flower essence you would receive from a practitioner or buy for immediate use in a store.

How They Work

Flower essences are vibratory, or energy, medicine and are intended to work primarily on mental/emotional states of mind and being. According to Dr. Bach, "Behind all disease lie our fears, our anxieties, our greed, our likes and dislikes." Bach believed that if negative states of mind and emotion can be transmuted into positive ones, "with the healing of them will go the disease from which we suffer." Although he discovered his remedies intuitively, Dr. Bach was a physician trained in the scientific tradition of Western medicine and did not declare a remedy effective unless it actually had a demonstrable and beneficial effect on patients to whom it was prescribed.

"This system of treatment is the most perfect which has been given to mankind within living memory," Bach modestly declared in his pamphlet, *The Twelve Healers and Other Remedies*. "It has the power to cure disease; and, in its simplicity, it may be used in the household." Bach encouraged people not only to use the essences, but to make them as well. In *The Seven Helpers* he states, "In this system of healing everything may be done by the people themselves, even, if they like, to the finding of the plants and the making of the remedies." *The Twelve Healers and Other Remedies,* now in its fifteenth printing, was self-published by Bach in 1933, and sold by him for 2 cents (when he remembered to charge for it!). The booklet contains detailed instructions for preparing flower essences according to his methods.

ARE FLOWER ESSENCES SAFE TO USE?

Absolutely. A "dosage" bottle of flower essence that you would receive from a practitioner or buy in a store is very dilute. Being a form of vibrational medicine, flower essences have no physical effects whatsoever, and consequently there are no physical side effects. Because they are harmless, they are particularly well suited for use with babies and children, with the elderly, even with pets and houseplants during times of illness and stress.

The art of prescribing flower essences rests on the ability to differentiate between various emotional and mental states, and sufficient knowledge of the essences themselves to know which are appropriate to use at what time. The best way to learn is to try them out and keep track of the results. Mothers, being intuitive and often very adept at discerning the thoughts and feelings of those within the family, tend to excel at this.

Start simply, by choosing one to three essences that address the problem at hand. Four to five drops of flower essence from the dosage bottle can be placed directly under the tongue or added to a small glass of water or juice, repeating the dose about every four hours. In emergency cases of intense emotion or mental turbulence, the essences can be given by mouth or rubbed on the inside of the wrist, administered as often as every fifteen minutes to an hour, as needed. Each person is unique, so it is difficult to know how long it will take to notice results. In some cases there will be an immediate response. Others may need to take a course of treatment for up to two weeks to see a change, at which point the remedy can be adjusted. If you administer the wrong flower essence, it simply won't bring about the desired result. If and when this happens, take a moment to reevaluate, try to understand what went wrong with your choice, and pick another suitable remedy.

While having the cooperation of the recipient is ideal, flower essences do not depend on the awareness of the individual being treated to have an effect. Nursing mothers can take flower essences themselves and have an effect on their infants. Flower essences can be added to the family water or beverage supply for their beneficial, harmonizing effects. Essences can be used in bathwater and added to lotions and creams. One practitioner I know dilutes them in a saline solution for use in eyedrops.

Flower essences can be a tremendous help to ease the emotional bumps and bruises of day-to-day family life, from bedtime fears to babysitter blues for children, from workplace stresses to relationship and life changes that accompany new parenthood for moms and dads. Every conceivable situation in life can be aided and eased by the gentle, balancing energy of flower essences. Because of the many hats I wear, at work and at home, I personally find myself turning to them for assistance in maintaining my emotional equilibrium nearly every day.

Dr. Bach and the Original Bach Flower Essences

Born in 1886, Edward Bach studied allopathic medicine and became a medical doctor in Great Britain in 1912. During his internship, Dr. Bach quickly noticed that conventional methods of treatment of the physical symptoms of disease often did not result in healing, especially in cases of chronic illness. Observation of patients in the ward led him to conclude that the personality of an individual had more to do with illness and disease than with the body. Searching for more effective, simpler, painless methods of treatment that were unavailable at the time, he became interested in immunology and began to work as a bacteriologist.

As a bacteriologist, Dr. Bach discovered a set of germs that he found in the intestines of patients suffering from chronic diseases which resisted standard medical treatment. He developed a vaccine from these intestinal bacteria, and as those inoculated were restored to a state of health, he also noticed a concurrent falling away of symptomatic complaints such as headaches, rheumatism, and arthritis. His success with the intestinal toxemia vaccination led him to study the connection between diet and disease, and later homeopathy, during his employment as pathologist and bacteriologist at the London Homeopathic Hospital.

Hahnemann, the founder of homeopathy, had discovered a century earlier the link between intestinal poisoning and chronic disease and had classified the poisons causing chronic illness into three categories. On studying Hahnemann's work, Dr. Bach recognized that the organisms he had found in the intestines were one and the same as the illness-causing poison Hahnemann had named "psora." Dr. Bach went on to develop seven homeopathic oral vaccines, or nosodes, which, when taken, resulted in the cleansing and restoration of the intestinal tract and digestive processes. As intestinal health was restored, overall health in his patients improved, and numerous symptoms disappeared without ever having been locally treated.

In line with Hahnemann's philosophy, Dr. Bach also believed that true healing involved treating the person and not the disease, and that disease is fundamentally spiritual in origin—the result of disharmony between the aims of the soul and the habits, thoughts, and desires of the personality. By restoring people to their true state of being—that of balance, happiness, and attunement to their particular soul purpose—Bach believed that physical ailments would cease to exist. Above all, he was dedicated to discovering an effective, pure, safe, simple, and inexpensive method of healing derived from nature that could be practiced by anyone.

Work on his own system of healing began in earnest with his recognition that there were twelve basic, or "world," types of personalities in the people he saw around him, and that each tended to react to any illness with a similar disturbance in mood and behavior. This realization only reinforced the concept that the patient, not the disease, must be treated. Following the advice of Paracelsus, Dr. Bach began to walk the pages of nature's textbook with his feet, spending long hours among the wild plants in the countryside of Wales. Working intuitively, he discovered the first three flower remedies and brought them back to London, where he prepared them according to homeopathic methods and prescribed them to various patients with good results.

Inspired by this success, in 1930, at the age of forty-three, Dr. Bach sold everything he owned, left London, his medical practice, and all his previous work and studies, and returned to Wales to focus exclusively on perfecting what would eventually become known as the Bach flower remedies. During that year, he changed from the homeopathic method of preparing the essences to the sun method, the discovery of which delighted him due to its simplicity and use of the four elements: "The earth to nurture the plant, the air from which it feeds, the sun or fire to enable it to impart its power, and water to collect and be enriched with its beneficent magnetic healing," as he described it.

Over the next few years, Dr. Bach discovered twelve basic flower essences to be used as remedies for the personality types he had perceived, and twenty-six "helper" remedies for transitory states of mind and feeling, for a total of thirty-eight. Having declared his work complete, he died in his sleep in 1936, two months after his fiftieth birthday.

∾

While I have tried a variety of flower essences made by a number of different companies over the years, I find myself returning time and again to the Bach flower remedies for day-to-day use. In my opinion, of the many flower essences available, the Bach remedies are the simplest, most direct, and easiest to understand. I prefer the original remedies, prepared by the methods established by Dr. Bach himself. These are currently available in health food stores and alternative pharmacies under the label "Healing Herbs" and are made with love and integrity by a husband-and-wife team who are also parents, Martine and Julian Barnard, in Wales.

In addition to the original Bach flower remedies, flower essences are now being made from Sierra and Rocky Mountain wildflowers, Himalayan flowers, cactus flowers, vegetables, old roses, and Peruvian orchids, to name just a few. They are made by people in the United States and all over the world, from California, Colorado, Alaska, and Hawaii to Africa, Europe,

Russia, Australia, and New Zealand. According to those who make them, these new essences are necessary to address a wide variety of subtle conditions that did not exist in Bach's time, such as protection from electromagnetic fields and environmental pollution. Many are made under auspicious astrological configurations, or in sacred places, such as the orchid essences made from flowers that grow near Machu Picchu in Peru. To illustrate the diversity of what is currently available, the Flower Essence Pharmacy on the Mendocino coast of California sells flower essences from forty-five different companies located in thirteen countries. (See the listing in the "Resource Guide.")

CHOOSING THE RIGHT FLOWER ESSENCE

Flower essences can be chosen based on observation of the intended recipient, or a conversation or interview with him or her. If a number of remedies are indicated, some practitioners will choose from among them intuitively, through use of a pendulum. For children, who may not always be articulate in describing their state of mind or feelings, I have found it useful to have them choose for themselves, by looking through photographs of the flowering plants from which the essences are made. This method, while also intuitive, can reveal inner states that even a mother may not be able to see.

The first time I did this with my ten-year-old son, I told him to pick one or more "favorites," pictures of flowers that looked especially beautiful to him. He picked all thirty-eight, saying the plants were all so beautiful he couldn't choose one over another! Generally, however, it's amazing to see how a child or adult tends to choose the exact remedy or combination of remedies she or he needs most, simply by looking at the photographs.

According to Nickie Murray, former trustee of the Bach Center and a longtime student of Dr. Bach's protégé, Nora Weeks, the original twelve Bach remedies are generally sufficient for treating children, whose mental and emotional states tend to be simpler and more direct than those of adults. The "helper" remedies are generally more appropriate for the complexities and transitory states of mind that accompany adulthood and the pressures of being out in the world. However, I have used a few of the "helpers" with my own children when the situation warranted, for example, honeysuckle and larch.

Making a Flower Essence—The Sun Method

Equipment: a clear glass bowl, spring water, sharp scissors (used only for this purpose), a camera loaded with film, a notebook and something to write or draw with, a tweezers, a funnel (preferably glass), a strainer (fine steel mesh or muslin cloth), a large, dark glass bottle to hold the finished essence, a label, brandy in a quantity equal to the amount of flower essence, labels, 2-ounce dark glass bottles with dropper tops for use as dosage bottles. (OPTIONAL: a magnifying glass, a local wildflower guide, tobacco or cornmeal to use as an offering)

Find the plants from which you wish to make an essence. Generally, they should be wild plants growing in a fairly pristine environment, rather than alongside a road or in a heavily traveled area. If you find wild plants on someone else's property, ask permission to use them, and reassure the owner that you will not be destroying the plant or removing it from the premises.

You may wish to spend some time in meditation and communication with the plants in advance of the day on which you make the essence, and ask them to help you ascertain the most propitious time for creating the flower essence. Not every plant is ready to be used when you are ready to make the essence! Respect the plant's right to say "no," or "not today." Sometimes flowers that are at their height of potency and are ready to be made into an essence will seem to have a glow about them, or to shout at you as you pass by.

If there is an abundance of plants of the same type and you are not sure which to use, ask for a sign or indication. I once went hiking to look for an appropriate place to make a mustard flower essence when the mustard plants were blooming all over the hillsides. There were so many plants in perfect bloom, how could I choose? Asking for a sign, I continued on my way and was surprised a short time later by the appearance of a young wild rabbit. Normally I do not get to see much more than the disappearing tail of a wild bunny. But this one let me walk right up, albeit quietly and carefully, within a few feet, where it remained for several minutes munching some greens that were growing . . . next to a patch of blooming mustard! Be sure to stay open to recognizing your sign when it appears.

When you have found the plant from which the essence will be made, you may wish to present it with an offering. Native

Americans have traditionally used cornmeal or tobacco. I have used these, and pennies or coins as well. The important thing is to acknowledge that the plant is giving you something of value, which gift you honor by giving something of value in return.

The best time of day to make a flower essence is when the sun is at the peak of its power, usually sometime between 11 A.M. and 3 P.M. Wear light-colored, comfortable clothing. If there is a natural spring near where the plants are growing, this is the ideal water to use to fill the bowl. If not, you'll have to bring your own.

Begin by preparing yourself. Make sure that you're in a peaceful, open state of mind. Do not try to make a flower essence when your thoughts or emotions are turbulent. Wait until your heart and mind are clear.

Use a clear glass bowl that has not been used previously for any other purpose. Dr. Bach destroyed his bowls after using them, but you might prefer to recycle yours for use in the kitchen.

Use new scissors that also have not been used for any other purpose. After sitting for a short time with the plants to establish a friendly connection, say a short prayer or blessing to set the tone of the spiritual atmosphere. You may wish to have another person with you to hold the bowl as you cut the most perfect of the plant's blooms. Do not touch the flowers! Let them fall directly onto the surface of the water in the bowl. When the surface is covered with a layer of blossoms, set the bowl on the earth in a place where it is in full contact with the sun's rays. Leave it this way for several hours, until you can see that the energy has left the flowers and transferred into the water. This is difficult to explain. I didn't understand how one could "see" an energy transference, but after having made my own essences, I can assure you that you *can* see it.

As you sit, waiting for the essence to be made, you can photograph the plant, examine it carefully, draw pictures of it, write about it, and otherwise become fully acquainted. Record your intuitive response to the plant. Note any physical aspects of the plant that might be related to its healing properties. Note colors, textures, shapes, aromas, number of petals, arrangement of leaves. Where is it growing? What is growing nearby? Sit with the plant as you would with a new friend, listening attentively, learning all that it is willing to reveal.

When the water is charged, remove the blossoms from the bowl with the tweezers. Put the funnel into the large bottle. Pour the flower essence through the strainer and into the bottle. Label your "mother tincture" with the name of the plant, the date, and the location. If there is any water left in the bowl, you can drink it, or use it to water the plant from which it came. If you drink it, be sure to monitor your own thoughts, feelings, and reactions that may be related to imbibing the flower essence.

When you get home, preserve the flower essence in an equal amount of brandy. To make a dosage bottle, almost fill a dark glass bottle with a dropper top with water. Add two or three drops of your flower essence mother tincture, and a little bit of brandy as a preservative. Shake gently. Doses of four to six drops can be given from this bottle as needed.

MOTHER EARTH'S TOP TWELVE BACH FLOWER REMEDIES: *THE TWELVE HEALERS*

Agrimony: For those who tend to hide their personal anguish behind a cheerful facade. Natural harmonizers and peace-lovers, Agrimony types will absorb much to avoid an argument and, as noted by Dr. Bach, may turn to drugs or alcohol to help them keep their spirits up. The remedy can help them to develop the kind of inner peace that cannot be disturbed by external events.

Centaury: The "doormat" remedy, for those who are too eager to serve others, even to their own detriment. Centaury types may attract troublesome relationships with bullies and dominating personalities that force them to come to terms with their own weaknesses. The remedy can help them begin to take a more active role in pursuit of their own life purpose, rather than passively serving the needs of others.

Cerato: Lack of trust in oneself, one's own opinion and inner voice. Being unduly influenced by others to one's detriment. This is an excellent remedy for children who are overly susceptible to peer pressure, who "go along" with a group, especially if doing so involves choices or activities that override their own good judgment, when they should "know better."

Chicory: Chicory types tend to be overprotective, clingy, or intrusively involved in the lives and affairs of friends and family. This is also a good remedy for the child who attempts to control parents' behavior with tantrums or illnesses, out of a desire to keep them close and within sight at all times.

Clematis: Clematis types suffer a lack of interest in present reality manifesting as dreaminess or living in a dream of the future. Clematis children may miss their lessons at school due to too much daydreaming. The remedy helps bring dreamy, unfocused types down to earth, and is also used for comatose or semiconscious states.

Gentian: Gentian types are those who are too quick to give up and are too easily discouraged or disheartened. Life presents them with an obstacle, and instead of responding to the challenge, they fold. Gentian can also be used for temporary feelings of defeat, for encouragement, and strengthening of purpose or resolve.

Impatiens: Impatient, quick-tempered, and quick-thinking people who prefer to work alone and at their own speed. Impatiens types have very little patience with being ill. Their angry outbursts may be disconcerting to those around them, but such moods tend to be superficial and not intentionally malicious in nature, caused by frustration with those who, in their estimation, are not "up to speed." The remedy Impatiens can help them to develop greater tolerance and compassion.

Mimulus: For everyday fears that can be described, such as fear of the dark, fear of being left alone, fear of animals or strangers, fear of things that are known. Mimulus types do not easily share their fears with others, but tend to keep them inside, although they may manifest physical symptoms. This is a wonderful remedy for children who are too shy, and can be useful on occasions such as the first day of school, before taking tests, at parties, before the arrival of babysitters, and before doctor or dentist visits.

Rock Rose: For traumatic fear or terror, such as that resulting from accidents, assaults, natural disasters or catastrophes, or sudden illness. This is a remedy to use in the aftermath of car accidents, earthquakes, tornadoes, floods, and hurricanes, before surgery, during an asthmatic attack, or for any condition that engenders deep fear of death or bodily harm.

Scleranthus: Indecisiveness, the inability to choose or distinguish the better of two things. The Scleranthus type, while agonizing over making the choice, suffers in quiet solitude, not seeking the advice of others to aid in making the decision.

Vervain: Strong, confident, organized proselytizers who continually attempt to convert others to their own cherished beliefs or points of view. The remedy can help them to gently accept the differences of others, and to keep their own opinions to themselves until asked.

Water Violet: Water Violets tend to be aloof, quiet, and independent. Often very talented or intelligent, they mind their own business and prefer their own company to that of others. Because they are so self-reliant, they may be lonely without even realizing it. Water Violet was grouped by Dr. Bach under the remedies for loneliness.

BACH FLOWER REMEDIES: *THE TWENTY-SIX HELPERS*

Aspen: For a state of dread, of fear without a known cause, the inexplicable feeling that something terrible is going to happen.

Beech: For those who tend to be intolerant and critical of everything and everyone around them, to help them "see more good and beauty," as Dr. Bach put it.

Cherry Plum: For fear of losing control, having a breakdown, or committing desperate acts. Thoughts of violence against others or suicidal tendencies. While this is not a remedy one would normally consider for a child, but under certain circumstances it may be necessary.

Chestnut Bud: For those who do not learn by observation of themselves, others, or life and who therefore tend to make the same mistakes over and over again. This remedy aids in recognizing our spiritual lessons when life presents them to us.

Crab Apple: The cleansing remedy. For those who miss the big picture because they are so fussily focused on some small detail.

For those who feel unclean, or as if they have come into contact with something poisonous, impure, or unclean.

Elm: For the temporary feeling of being overwhelmed, in those who are otherwise very capable and fulfilling their true soul's mission in life. For the feeling that the tasks they have taken on in life are beyond their power to accomplish or are unachievable. Elm reminds us to keep the light of joy alive in our hearts as we strive to make the world a better place.

Gorse: For hopelessness. The belief that nothing more can be done about an illness or negative situation. Gorse helps to keep the ray of hope alive, no matter how difficult the circumstance.

Heather: The chatterbox remedy, for those who cannot stand to be alone and are forever telling others—family, friends, or complete strangers—about themselves and their problems. Heather encourages inner peace and tranquillity.

Holly: For troublesome attacks of envy, jealousy, suspicion, or revenge. This remedy helps increase feelings of love and compassion, thereby lessening attacks of "vexation" that create the negative Holly state. Kathy Arnos, in her booklet *Bach Flowers for Children,* suggests Holly for sibling rivalry.

Honeysuckle: Living in the past, with a belief that the present and future hold no real happiness that can compare with past experiences. This remedy encourages us to forget the past, go for the gusto, plunge into the present. It can be useful for children of separated or divorced parents, especially those who continue to wish (for years, sometimes) that their parents will reunite, or who idealize the life they had before their parents split up.

Hornbeam: The (temporary) feeling that one hasn't the strength or ability, mentally or physically, to do what needs to be done, often resulting in procrastination. It's all just "too much." Hornbeam helps restore enthusiasm for the task at hand.

Larch: For low self-esteem. Lack of confidence and feelings of inadequacy create a self-fulfilling prophecy of failure. The message of Larch is to remind us that we cannot help but succeed, for we are all the invincible children of God.

Mustard: Sudden, inexplicable gloom, described by Dr. Bach "as though a cold, dark cloud overshadowed them and hid the light and joy of life." The remedy restores the soul's true state of being, which is one of joy, happiness, and peace.

Oak: Strong, brave people who keep going against all odds but who may take on too much. Those who may not realize their own limits until they reach the breaking point. Oak teaches us to stop struggling against our faults and shortcomings and to focus instead on cultivating our virtues.

Olive: For exhaustion and weariness, mental or physical, such as is experienced after a long struggle or illness, in which even the smallest day-to-day tasks seem to be too much. Olive helps to restore the perfect balance of body, mind, and spirit that is the foundation of true health.

Pine: For guilt. For those who blame themselves for everything, whether or not it was actually their fault, and who are never content with what they do or have done, no matter how hard they have tried. The remedy reminds us of our own inherent perfection.

Red Chestnut: For fear that something horrible might happen to other people or to loved ones. The remedy restores perspective, allowing us to be loving and sympathetic toward others without being consumed by anxiety over their welfare.

Rock Water: For the uptight ascetic who tends toward self-denial and may be overly obsessed with setting a good example, especially in the moral or spiritual realms. Rock Water helps us to realize that true spirituality is a joyful state of being, not just a set of strict rules to be followed.

Star of Bethlehem: For shock or inconsolable grief. Star of Bethlehem brings spiritual comfort, the biblical state of "peace which passeth understanding."

Sweet Chestnut: For heartbreak and intense, unbearable anguish of the heart, the "dark night of the soul." The remedy reminds us that we are never given a spiritual challenge greater than our capacity to bear.

Vine: For those ultra-capable, domineering persons who tend to control or direct all those around them. Vine helps us to allow others to be free to be themselves and follow their own soul's path.

Walnut: For protection from outside influences that pull us away from pursuit of our ambitions, goals, and ideals. The remedy also lends protection during times of transition, reevaluation, or life changes, such as marriage, parenthood, or divorce.

White Chestnut: For the overactive mind, in which unwanted, undesired thoughts or ideas interfere with focusing on present activities. Lack of inner peace due to turbulent, worrisome, even meaningless repetitive thoughts that will not go away. White Chestnut helps restore inner peace and quiet.

Wild Oat: For uncertainty as to one's true calling in life. Undirected ambition and the inability to choose a focus from among many interests and possibilities. Wild Oat helps us to recognize and assume our own unique niche in the grand scheme of things.

Wild Rose: For resignation. Those who stop making any effort to change or improve their lives, who live with a kind of joyless inertia. The remedy can help to restore a sense of adventure.

Willow: For resentment of the trials and struggles of life, and for those who feel they do not deserve the hand they've been dealt in life, and thus become bitter and blame others, or circumstances. The lesson of Willow is cheerful acceptance of our place in life.

The medical school of the future will not particularly interest itself in the ultimate results and products of disease, nor will it pay so much attention to actual physical lessons, or administer drugs and chemicals merely for the sake of palliating our symptoms, but knowing the true cause of sickness and aware that the obvious physical results are merely secondary, it will concentrate its efforts upon bringing about that harmony between body, mind and soul which results in the relief and cure of disease. And in such cases as are undertaken early enough the correction of the mind will avert the imminent illness.

—Dr. Edward Bach, *Heal Thyself*

CHAPTER FIVE

AROMATHERAPY

The Sweet Breathing of Flowers

*The voice of the Great Spirit is heard
in the twittering of birds,
the rippling of mighty waters,
and the sweet breathing of flowers.*

—Gertrude Simmons Bonin, Zitkala-Sa (1876–1938)

he first essential oil I used with my own children was lavender, which I reached for one night instead of Tylenol to bring down a fever in my then four-year-old son. I had been using aromatherapy on myself to alleviate stress and enhance relaxation following a move back to the big city after a couple of idyllic years of living in a small mountain community. Although I had read a few books on the subject, I had yet to try aromatherapy on my children. At that point, I had no idea of how genuinely useful and effective essential oils could be.

I put a few drops of a fine French lavender essence in a tub of tepid water, then added my son to the bath. He was not a happy child as I poured the scented water over his chest, shoulders, and back. But after fifteen minutes, his temperature dropped dramatically. A few days later, his younger sister came down with a similar fever. Once again I used lavender, with the same results. I was so impressed I became an aromatherapy proselyte, pressing little bottles of lavender essence into the hands of every mother I encountered. I started using lavender for everything: insect bites, burns, stress relief for myself, calming the kids at bedtime. I took classes and became certified, and bought all the massage oils, bath gels, and essential oils I could find.

With education, it quickly became apparent to me that the word *aromatherapy* on the label did not necessarily mean there were therapeutic-grade essential oils present inside the bottle. Particularly suspicious were inexpensive grocery store items that claimed "aromatherapy." Having bought real essential oils, I was aware of their price, and of the short supply of genuine, untampered with essences appropriate for aromatherapeutic use. Also listed among the ingredients were alleged "essential oils" that I knew did not exist, such as "white ginger" and "gardenia." Just because something smells pleasant doesn't mean it qualifies as aromatherapy, no matter what the label says.

WHAT IS AROMATHERAPY?

True aromatherapy is much more than just a pretty smell! In fact, many of the hundreds of essential oils available today don't smell "pretty" at all. You would never dab essence of tea tree, for example, behind your ears before an evening out, yet it is one of the most studied, useful, and versatile aromatic essences. Simply defined, aromatherapy is the use of essential oils derived from plants for purposes of encouraging the well-being of body, mind, and spirit.

Essential oils are intensely concentrated natural essences obtained from fragrant leaves, roots, barks, flowers, and seeds using a number of different processes. Steam or water distillation is the most commonly used method for producing essential oils from herbs, for example, lavender, rosemary, or thyme, and flowers whose essences are sturdy enough to survive it, such as rose. Cold pressing is the preferred method for citrus fruits, from which the volatile essence is extracted by pressing the peel. Solvent extraction is generally limited to flowers such as jasmine, or tuberose, whose delicate essences would be destroyed by the heat and pressure of the distillation process. Carbon dioxide is also used for purposes of extraction, mostly for spice essences such as black pepper or nutmeg.

The term *aromatherapy* was coined in 1928 by the French cosmetic chemist René-Maurice Gattefossé, who became fascinated with the healing potential of essential oils after he successfully used lavender to cure serious burns he suffered in a laboratory explosion. Since the nineteenth century, research on the medical and psychotherapeutic applications of essential oils has been published in Europe, Australia, Japan, Russia, Egypt, and the United States. During World War II, a French army surgeon who was influenced by Gattefossé, Dr. Jean Valnet, used essential oils for treating battlefield injuries when supplies of penicillin ran short. Later, Dr. Valnet also used essential oils to treat psychiatric patients, with remarkable results. In 1964 he published his book *Aromatherapie*, still an excellent guide to medical applications of essential oils and their effectiveness against specific bacteria and pathogens.

A Brief History of Aromatics

The roots of aromatherapy as an art and a science extend as far back in human history to the earliest existing records of ancient Egypt and the Ayurvedic medicine of India. In ancient times there were no arbitrary divisions placed between the various levels of being. The same aromatics used to cure and prevent disease in the body were also used to influence mood and emotion and to communicate with and worship the divine.

Alexandria was the cultural hub of the ancient world, and it was there that the first still, used for distillation of aromatics, was developed by a female alchemist, Maria Prophetissima. Aromatic secrets and traditions radiated outward from their birthplace in ancient Egypt to the developing cultures of Greece and Rome. Theophrastus of Greece, the first aromatherapist and school friend of Alexander the Great, who sent Theophrastus botanical specimens of fragrant plants from his sojourns, wrote what is purported to be the first book on aromatherapy, titled *Concerning Odors*. The health- and aesthetic-minded Greeks continued to develop the arts of aromatic bathing and massage, habits that were picked up and fully indulged in by the pleasure-loving Romans. By the year 3 A.D., Rome housed thousands of many-chambered baths, the largest and most luxurious of which were a kind of combination modern-day shopping mall and athletic field, with stores, restaurants, game areas, swimming pools, and *unctuaria*, wherein the multistage bathing experience was finished off with a fragrant massage. Precious rose water ran in Roman fountains and was used for a variety of health purposes. The

Romans were extremely fond of roses and their decorative and medicinal uses. At one point there were so many acres of land outside Rome dedicated to the cultivation of roses that some worried about possible grain shortages.

By the time the Roman Empire fell, its conquering armies had disseminated Roman influence and habits to its farthest-flung reaches. Even during the Dark Ages in Europe, cloistered monks guarded many of the herbal and aromatic healing traditions that had been popular in earlier times. The same roses once cultivated over thousands of acres outside Rome were now carefully tended in walled monastery gardens. Medicinal liqueurs distilled by contemplative nuns and monks preserved the secret healing recipes. Meanwhile, civilization blossomed in the Middle East, where perfumery and distillation reached new heights. The spice trade flourished, and the Crusaders returned, not with the Holy Grail in hand, but with "all the perfumes of Araby."

Throughout the eighteenth century, "spices" and aromatics were still being used for their aesthetic appeal, for flavoring, and as medicine. Many preparations, especially those made with alcohol, were used internally as medicinal tonics as well as externally as perfumes or friction rubs. Napoleon, for example, used more than six hundred bottles of cologne per year, a blend of antiseptic and healing aromatic essences including rosemary, mint, thyme, and sage in a natural alcohol base. The diminutive emperor not only drank it; he splashed it on as a personal perfume and used it to cleanse and disinfect wounds incurred in battle as well.

In France during the late 1700s, perfumery and medicine were separated into two distinct categories. Perfumers focused exclusively on the aesthetic and emotional effects of blending, while the new medical doctors carved out a niche for their "scientific" practices by discrediting thousands of years of natural healing tradition. Ironically, aromatherapy has come full circle, as the healing powers of essential oils are being rediscovered and documented by modern medical research. France is now at the forefront of medical aromatherapy.

Aromatherapy Today

In the past, when the composition of essential oils was a mystery, even without understanding the chemical processes involved people were able to profit from their antiseptic properties whether in the form of food (garlic, onion, etc.) or vapours for the prevention and control of epidemics. Hippocrates, for instance, tackled the plague epidemic in Athens by fumigating the city with aromatic essences. In the nineteenth century, perfumery workers always showed an almost complete immunity during cholera outbreaks. This was forgotten in 1970 when panic raged throughout the Western world at the news of a few cases of cholera in the Near East. Some businessmen who escaped vaccination returned hale and hearty from the countries in question. [A]ll they had taken with them were charcoal tablets, magnesium—and essential oil drops.

—Jean Valnet, M.D., *The Practice of Aromatherapy*

All essential oils have healing properties and are antiseptic and bacteriostatic to a greater or lesser degree. In recent studies, essential oils and their chemical constituents have been documented to have a wide variety of effects on a broad spectrum of conditions.

More and more research is being done to investigate the potential for therapeutic use of essential oils in serious medical conditions. Some studies confirm traditional uses of the herbs from which essential oils are derived. Others are breaking new ground entirely. For example, the chemical constituents linalool and linalyl aldehyde, which are present in lavender essence, appear to have an inhibiting effect on nerve impulses, which may explain lavender's anesthetic and relaxing effects. Myristicin, a component of nutmeg oil, has been shown to have anti-inflammatory, antioxidant, and antitumoral effects and to increase brain serotonin, lower blood pressure, and function as an anti-depressant and sedative.

On the physical level, studies done in the 1950s and 1960s confirm that as aggressive as essential oils can be toward pathogenic microorganisms, they are harmless to healthy living tissue when used in proper dilution. This is not the case with many other chemicals that have been used for similar antiseptic or germicidal purposes. In a 1958 study, vapors derived from aromatic plants were shown to inhibit development of certain strains of *Staphylococcus* and coliform bacteria. In descending order of potency, the essential oils tested were thyme, rosemary, eucalyptus, peppermint, neroli, and pine.[1]

A French study conducted in 1963 found a vaporized antimicrobial blend of pine, thyme, peppermint, lavender, rosemary, cloves, and cinnamon to be very effective, destroying over 90 percent of the colonies of molds and bacteria, such as *Staphylococci,* that were present in the room before the spray was used.[2] The same combination of essences used in another study three years earlier had been shown to prevent the spread of pathogens causing infectious childhood diseases such as whooping cough, nasal catarrh, and influenza, as well as respiratory diseases such as flu, tuberculosis, and pneumonia in adults. Day care centers, those notorious vectors of nasty cold and flu germs that preschoolers carry home to parents and family members, should, in my opinion, all be diffusing such a blend!

Aromatherapy is being used to improve the sleep patterns of hospital and nursing home patients and to reduce the amount of night sedation they require. Essential oils have also been shown to reduce stress levels in coronary care patients. A study of 122 patients admitted to a general intensive care unit was described as resulting in "significantly greater improvement in their mood and perceived levels of anxiety" for those who were given aromatherapy, specifically the essential oil of lavender. A 1996 study of myrrh conducted by researchers at the University of Florence confirmed the resin's aromatherapeutic reputation as an analgesic.[3]

Essential oils are also being studied for their possible anticarcinogenic effects. D-limonene, a terpene found in citrus oils such as lime and lemon, is being studied for its effectiveness in reducing and preventing tumors and breast cancer. Oral limonene has been used in a trial of pancreatic and colorectal cancer patients at Charing Cross Hospital in London. Perillyl alcohol, a monoterpene produced by lavender flowers, has been studied since 1982 at the University of Wisconsin Comprehensive Cancer Center in Madison for its apparent ability to cause regression of breast, liver, and pancreatic tumors in laboratory animals, and for its encouraging effects against leukemia. The Royal London Homeopathic Hospital uses aromatherapy as part of its Integrated Care Programme for Patients Living with Cancer. Essential oil of grapefruit, which gives grapefruit juice its bitter taste, was shown in a 1995 study to boost the potency of the antirejection drug Cyclosporine.[4]

Maria Lis-Balchin and Stanley Deans have investigated the activity of some fifty essential oils in inhibiting the growth of twenty-five bacteria and fungi species.[5] This group is also looking into the antioxidant properties of essences such as thyme, marjoram, oregano, sage, and rosemary.[6] Recent research shows that two components of rosemary essential oil, carnosol and carnosic acid, may function as antioxidants, helping to protect cells and tissues from damage.[7] Citral, found in steam-distilled essences of rose and lemongrass, has antiseptic and possibly viricidal properties. According to Indian research, jasmone, a chemical component of *Jasminum grandiflorum*, appears to be effective in the treatment of hepatitis and cirrhosis, and to aid in pain control.[8] Essential oils have also been used to condition immune response, thereby reducing the need for medication.

Through use of essential oils in diffusers and massage, nurses are integrating aromatherapy to create a more nurturing environment and to ease chronic conditions such as chronic pain and inflammation, arthritis, mood disorders, depression, Alzheimer's disease, and skin disorders. Lavender, clary sage, jasmine, peppermint, rose, tea tree and ylang-ylang essential oils have been administered through massage and inhalation at the Intensive Care Unit at Royal Berkshire and Battle hospitals in the United Kingdom. There a controlled study of the physiologically measurable effects of massage with a 1 percent dilution of lavender essence yielded dubious results, although the patients themselves reported a perceived benefit in terms of anxiety and stress reduction.[9] Aromatherapy case studies reported by practitioners in the *International Journal of Aromatherapy* include a multitude of diverse conditions, from PMS and eczema to bedwetting and Hodgkin's disease.

Anne Boyle, now associate dean of the School of Dental Medicine at Southern Illinois University, conducted a controlled study at the Case Western Reserve University School of Dentistry that found positive results from using essential oils for reducing stress and anxiety levels in dental patients about to undergo root canals. The study, reported in the March 1996 issue of *Aromatic Thymes,* inspired Dr. Boyle to continue her research into the benefits of aromatherapy, and she is currently performing research into the physiological effects of essential oils on anxiety by measuring blood pressure, heart rate, galvanic skin response, temperature changes, and brain waves.[10]

Daniel Penoel and Daniel Lapraz continue their ongoing pioneering work with medical and psychiatric applications of essential oils. Tim Betts, a British neuropsychiatrist, has experimented with essential oils of lavender, chamomile, ylang-ylang, geranium, rosemary, and lemongrass in aromatherapy massage for patients with epilepsy.

Aromatherapy research may also hold intriguing possibilities for those of us approaching middle age and our later years. Dietary thyme oil has been shown to raise levels of polyunsaturated fatty acids, which may have a preventive effect on aging and such conditions as senile dementia. British researchers at Newcastle General Hospital in northern England found that sage essential oil inhibits the activity of an enzyme believed to play a role in the memory loss that characterizes Alzheimer's disease.[11]

How to Use Essential Oils

Essential oils can enter the body through inhalation, ingestion, or absorption through the skin during a bath or massage. The essences then enter the bloodstream and circulate through the body for several hours before being excreted. The route they take out of the body is often related to the essence's healing effects. Sandalwood, for instance, is used for genitourinary system problems and is secreted through those pathways. Eucalyptus is known for its effectiveness in improving respiratory function and leaves the body through the breath. Because they are not retained in tissues or fat, essential oils have virtually no side effects when properly applied. And, remarkably, bacteria and germs do not develop resistance to essential oils the way they do with pharmaceutical antibiotics.

I do not recommend taking essential oils internally without the guidance of a qualified medical practitioner. In Europe, where doctors and nurses prescribe essential oils and aromatherapy is covered by medical insurance, the essences are sold alongside pharmaceutical drugs. In this country, the situation is very different. For home use, I recommend staying with external applications, such as the diffuser, bath, or shower, or, the most effective of all, aromatherapy massage.

A diffuser can be as simple as a ceramic lightbulb ring or as complex as the professional practitioner's diffusing machine, which includes an air pump that breaks the essence up into a fine "nebulized" mist. The lightbulb heats the ceramic ring and causes the essence to volatilize and disperse through the air, where it can then be inhaled. The chief benefit of this method is its simplicity. However, heating the essence can cause chemical changes that may affect its therapeutic potency. (Lightbulb rings made of metal get too hot for essential oils.) Heat is also the main drawback of the potpourri-type diffuser, in which a few drops of essential oil are added to a small bowl of heated water placed above a light-bulb or candle. Essential oils added to the medicament well of a steam vaporizer can be effective for alleviating coughs and conges-tion that accompany colds and flu. While the heat methods scent the air effectively, the health benefits of the diffusing machine are believed by many aromatherapists to be superior. In addition, as the molecules of essential oil settle on surfaces such as furniture and floors, they continue their disinfecting action.

For general preventive purposes and for keeping the air clean while someone in the house is ill, try the following diffuser blends: lavender, eucalyptus, and tea tree; orange and cinnamon; lavender and clove; thyme, lavender, and lemon. Diffuser blends should be made with pure, undiluted essential oils only.

Essential oils can also be used effectively in the bath. The mildest essences, such as lavender or rose, can be dropped directly into the water and dispersed just before stepping in. (Don't add them while the water is still running, or the oils will evaporate before you've entered the tub!) Essences can also be mixed with a tablespoon of diluent, such as milk, oil, liquid soap or bath gel, before being added to the tub, to help them disperse more evenly through the water. Dilution is especially effective with oils that have the potential to irritate the skin, such as rosemary, eucalyp-tus, or thyme (except for the mild linalol chemotype of the latter), and with hydrophobic essences that don't mix well with water, such as blue chamomile.

CARE AND STORAGE OF ESSENTIAL OILS

Pure essential oils are packaged in small dark glass bottles with dropper tops, and should be stored out of direct sunlight and away from heat sources or great temperature variations. Floral waters and hydrolates, which are by-products of the distillation process, should be kept in the refrigerator, which is where I also keep some of my more delicate essences, such as carrot seed oil, and perishable carriers such as Rosa Mosqueta or evening prim-rose oil. Keep essential oils out of the reach of children.

The essential oil market is volatile (no pun intended!), and pricing will vary widely, based on availability and preciousness of the oil. For example, tea tree, usually a medium-priced oil, became very expensive and hard to find following bad weather in Australia that destroyed much of the crop. Rare and precious essences such as rose, melissa, jasmine, and neroli, as well as some of the more obscure absolutes and concretes used in perfumery, will always be expensive. Organic essential oils generally cost a bit more, as will any "specialty" oil. Citrus oils will be on the low end of the price spectrum, due to the abundant production of citrus crops here in the United States, although specialty citrus essences from other countries such as Italy and Israel will be more costly due to the limited amount available. Generally, cold-pressed citrus essences are more effective for aromatherapy than those that are steam dis-tilled, which tend to be used more for flavoring.

CHOOSING AND USING AN ESSENCE

When choosing an essence, let your nose be your guide. Studies have shown that more often than not, the essential oil that smells good to you is the essence that you need. Refine your sensibilities by training your olfactory system to respond to the highest-quality essences you can find. Look for the botanical name and country of origin on the label, and always smell before you buy. There's a beauty and wholesomeness about the aroma of a high-quality essence. Don't be fooled by lower-priced, low-grade essential oils, which are basically a waste of time and money. They may be fine to use for scenting candles or potpourri, but they will not perform satisfactorily in an aromatherapeutic sense. Good-quality essential oils are eminently worth the investment. A drop or two of a high-grade oil will outperform bottles of the poorer substitutes.

Be careful to avoid contact with eyes, genitals, and mucous membranes when using essential oils. Although quite safe to use when the appropriate oil is selected and blended in the proper dilution, essential oils can still cause irritation to sensitive tissues. If you're uncertain, perform a patch test by using a small amount of appropriately diluted essence on the skin of the arm, inside the elbow, and leave it on for a few hours. If you experience skin irritation, choose a different oil or increase the dilution.

If you don't get the results you want with the essence or combination you have chosen, try again. Every situation and every person is unique. When essential oils are used medicinally in Europe, a culture is taken of the microorganism associated with the discomfort or disease, and a number of different essences are then introduced to determine which most effectively inhibits the germ's or bacteria's growth. Such testing recognizes that there are many different strains of pathogens, and each will respond somewhat differently. A variety of essences can generally be used to alleviate any given condition. Be willing to experiment until you get the results you desire.

TOUCH AND SMELL

Touch is our first sense to develop. Touch is our connection to life and is essential to life from embryo to old age. Touch given from the heart in a joyful, respectful way is healing. Without a doubt, it is the most powerful form of communication.

—Teresa Ramsey, *Baby's First Massage*

Touch and smell are intricately related from the very beginning of life. A man and woman are attracted to each other through a complex interaction of personal aromas and pheromones that communicate their biological compatibility. The woman's reproductive cycle is stimulated into activity by the scent of the male. This at-first-distant molecular exchange draws them closer and creates a biochemical state that both urges and desires physical contact. Once touch occurs, even more attractant aromas are released, culminating in the most intimate form of touch, the sexual act. Then smell takes over once again as the sperm, it is believed, literally smells its way to the egg, which gives off a kind of come-hither perfume.

In utero, touch continues to stimulate development as the growing fetus comes into contact with the uterine walls. Before birth, the nasal passages are blocked with mucous plugs, which a recent film I saw labeled "of unknown purpose," although I personally believe the plugs are there to ensure that "primary olfactory memory," which is an integral part of the parent/child bonding process, does not happen prematurely. According to Michael Leon, professor of psychology at the University of

California at Irvine, "primary olfactory memory," which character-izes and bonds our closest relationships, is established in as little as ten minutes following birth. However, olfactory bonding must be reinforced with touch at the same time, or the newborn's "bonding" memory will not be permanently etched in the brain. It is the combination of touch and smell that anchors our first and deepest bonding experience. This, Dr. Leon believes, is nature's way of making sure that infants don't bond with just any old smell floating by.[12]

This is also why the hours following birth are such an impor-tant time for parents and newborns to be together, a basic human requirement that is not always honored in the standard hospital birth experience. I have experienced a "normal" hospital birth, a vaginal delivery accompanied by fetal monitoring and an epidural with my first child, and subsequently a fairly drugged but con-scious "C-section" hospital birth with my second. While their dad was "allowed" to be present and to cut the cord both times, within minutes after both deliveries my babies were taken from me, and I was shunted off by myself to "recover," according to hospital routine. Comparing these experiences with the natural homebirth of my third child, assisted by a wonderful team of midwives who insisted that mother, father, and baby be left alone together for hours afterward, I am firmly convinced that while medical science can be a lifesaver for a mother and infant under-going abnormal complications, the majority of women, however we may have been conditioned to believe otherwise, do not require the intervention of doctors or technology to give birth. In my opinion, the inappropriate application of drugs and machin-ery in normal labors not only causes many of the complications cited to justify their use but also actively interferes with the normal bonding processes between parents and child and slows down the mother's recovery.

During birth, the pressure of uterine contractions and the pas-sage down the birth canal give the wake-up call to a newborn's life support systems, preparing the baby for the increased demands of life outside the womb. After birth, touching, cuddling, and contact with the mother's body provide continued stimulation to the infant's respiratory, cardiovascular, digestive, and immune systems. Skin to skin contact and the baby's nursing stimulate the mother's uterus to contract back to its prepregnancy size. Birth is a momen-tous experience on all levels, for all involved. Mother, father, and newborn need to be in close contact physically, emotionally, and spiritually for optimal familial bonding to occur.

Positive touch experiences are crucial to the healthy development of infants and children. How we are touched as we are growing up not only affects our perception of whether or not we are loved and how safe a place the world is; it also determines many aspects of our personality, our ability to relate to others, and the overall state of our health by influencing our biochemical makeup. Negative touch experiences are linked with failure to thrive in infants and children, stunted growth, emotional problems, inability to relate or empathize with others, and increased tendencies toward violence and drug abuse during adolescence.

AROMATHERAPY MASSAGE

Being touched and caressed,
being massaged,
is food for the infant.
Food as necessary
As minerals, vitamins, and proteins.
Deprived of this food,
the name of which is love,
babies would rather die.
And they often do.

—Frederick Leboyer, *Loving Hands*

I believe wholeheartedly in the benefits of massage, from infancy on through to the last moments of life. Studies show that babies who are lightly massaged have fewer respiratory problems and less vomiting and diarrhea. They cry less, smile and laugh more often, and breathe more deeply, which oxygenates the blood and helps circulation to newly functioning organs. Touch is also integral to brain development, as a recent study at the Baylor College of Medicine has shown. Researchers there found that children who are rarely touched have smaller brains, as much as 20 to 30 percent smaller than others their age who receive adequate stimulation.[13]

Infant massage originated thousands of years ago in the East, particularly in India and Pakistan, where there are written records of its practice that are more than three thousand years old. The benefits of infant massage extend beyond what can be attributed to physical contact. In a recent study conducted by researchers at the University of Miami School of Medicine's Touch and Research Institute, forty one- to three-month-old infants were either rocked or given a full body massage by researchers trained in infant massage for fifteen minutes, twice a week. The massaged infants gained more weight, were more alert when awake and fell asleep faster, were more easily soothed, and had lower levels of stress hormones than the babies who were only rocked.[14]

For older children, massage promotes body awareness and healthy muscle and tissue development, which encourages good posture and enhances participation in sports, gymnastics, and dance. Massage is also useful in children and adults for reducing stress and enhancing emotional stability and immune response. Self-esteem and self-confidence are also improved. In another Miami Touch and Research Institute study, fifty-two children and adolescents hospitalized for depression and adjustment disorder were given a daily half-hour back massage. Compared to a control group who had watched relaxing videotapes, the massaged kids slept better, were less anxious and more cooperative, and had lower levels of stress hormones.[15]

The addition of aromatherapy can make massage an even more powerful healing experience. One randomized controlled study, reported in a 1994 issue of *Complementary Therapies in Medicine,* found "statistically significant, lasting psychological benefit" for postcardiac surgery patients with foot massage using neroli, an essential oil derived from the blossom of the bitter orange, over massage with plain vegetable oil.[16] A 1995 study reported in the same journal claims an 80 percent success rate in benefiting cancer patients with the use of aromatherapy massage.[17] On a personal note, I recently received a moving letter from a mother whose daughter is suffering from childhood leukemia. After a long day of chemotherapy and other invasive treatments the child endures as she fights this deadly disease, aromatherapy massage at bedtime helps her to go to sleep at night and gives the mother at least one small thing she can do to help her daughter feel a bit better.

The beneficial effects of aromatherapy massage can also be enhanced by combining it with meditation and prayer in the form of directed healing intention. Thai medical tradition contains an excellent example of this. Influenced by both the Ayurvedic tradition of India and traditional Chinese medicine, Nuad Bo'Rarn, the traditional physical medicine of Thailand, is a form of healing massage that emphasizes the importance of *both* recipient and practitioner being in a meditative state during the massage. This healing massage is considered to be a practical application of the spiritual concept of Metta, or loving kindness. Emphasizing the mind/body connection, this 2,500-year-old tradition begins with a prayer by the practitioner, focusing on a clear and sincere intention to affect the physiology and vital energy of the body and mind of the recipient. In addition to treating physical ailments, Nuad Bo'Rarn, which is taught and practiced in Buddhist temples, is also used in Thailand to treat emotional and spiritual disorders.

Following are some healing massage techniques for you to try. For best results, take a few moments to center yourself and clarify your healing intentions before you begin. As you give a massage, also give the gift of your full presence, observing the response of the recipient and keeping your intuition tuned. If you detect signs of discomfort, adjust your actions accordingly. In terms of being touched, babies and children are just as individual as adults and have differing levels of tolerance and enjoyment. Some are automatically trusting and will relax completely, going into a receptive mode right from the very start. Others may have to be approached gradually, a few minutes at a time. Those who have had negative touch experiences may have the most difficult time accepting massage. With such babies, children, or adults, a simple foot massage is noninvasive and gives the benefits of healing touch while respecting boundaries and allowing for the gradual rebuilding of trust.

When using essential oils in a massage blend, both the giver and receiver of the massage derive aromatherapeutic benefit as the aroma is inhaled and essences are absorbed through the hands. According to Eastern traditions, energy meridians that carry vital forces throughout the body all terminate in the hands and feet, so that the massage you are giving is also a healing benefit you receive as you stimulate your own energy points.

Traditional Massage
for the Baby and Young Child

For thousands of years it has been traditional in India, as well as in related cultures such as those of Pakistan and Bali, for mothers to massage their babies. Indian women give their infants a ten- to fifteen-minute massage in the morning and in the evening, from the time the baby is one month old until it reaches the age of six months. Older babies and children may also be massaged, although the twice-daily routine is focused on the period that precedes the infant's mobility.

Most infant and young child massage currently being taught in this country is based on the ancient Indian routine handed down from mother to mother. If possible, be in contact with our own primordial mother, Mother Earth, drawing strength and serenity from her as the massage is given. In warm weather, spread a blanket over a sunny spot in the grass. Remove the baby's clothing and diaper, and put a towel over your lap to absorb any "spills." Babies and little ones chill easily, so have a light blanket on hand to cover them up if there's a breeze or if the temperature drops. Children should not be massaged right after eating. After a warm bath or just before naptime when they tend to be more relaxed can be a good time for a massage.

The following routine is for babies who are at least one month old. The remnant of the umbilical cord should have fallen off, and the navel area healed.

To begin, warm an ounce of oil, to which a drop of lavender, rose, chamomile, or mandarin essential oil has been added. The base oil should be a pure, cold-pressed vegetable or nut oil. Sesame, sweet almond, coconut, or safflower are all good choices. In cooler weather, the oil can be warmed briefly on the stove or in a potpourri-type burner. Just make sure it doesn't get too hot, or the oil may burn and the essence will evaporate. Make sure that your hands are clean and warm when you begin and that your nails are trimmed down. The baby or child should be laying on his or her back, feet toward you and facing up, as the massage begins. Laying a small baby on or between your legs affords a feeling of security. If the baby is fidgety, try wearing a pair of bright-patterned socks, which can serve to hold an infant's visual attention, especially if you wiggle your toes!

Rub a small amount of the blended oil between your palms to

warm it. Use just enough oil to allow your hands to slide freely along the child's skin. Do not use oil when massaging a child's hands or face, to prevent it from getting into the eyes.

The maintenance of a feeling connection is crucial if the massage is to be a healing experience for both of you and not just a superficial series of techniques. At first you'll be referring back and forth to the book and the massage may progress a bit awkwardly. But after a few sessions, you'll realize that there are only a few strokes to learn, and they make perfect sense physically, so that your hands will easily remember them. Gentle touch and healing intention are more important than perfect technique. No professional, no matter how well trained, can give your child or infant what you can give in the course of a healing massage, which is the gift of a parent's love expressed in a way that even a tiny baby can fully understand. Healing touch is a form of loving communication that travels to the deepest levels of being, to places where words cannot go. Gentle massage celebrates your child's beauty and perfection and keeps you "in touch" (literally) with the physical and behavioral changes that accompany growth and development. When I give a massage to my four-month-old infant the morning after giving a bedtime back rub or leg rub to my seven-year-old daughter or ten-year-old son, I am awed by the changes that can take place in the short span of a decade. They really do grow up so fast! The squirmy little jelly roll stretches out into the lean, lithe body of the preadolescent, with hints of the adult shape to come. What a joy, a pleasure, and a privilege it is to watch your children grow up straight and strong.

1. CHEST. Gently place your hands on the child's chest, and silently ask for permission to begin. This is an intuitive process and requires that you connect with your little one on a feeling level. Often the baby or child will make eye contact with you and smile, which can definitely be interpreted as a yes answer. If the baby is hungry or overly fussy, the answer may be no and you'll have to try another time.

2. CHEST. Now, using both hands in a smooth motion, move them outward from the center of the chest along the ribs and to the sides of the child's body, as if smoothing down the pages of a book. Repeat several times, slowly and gently.

3. CHEST. In this stroke, the hands move from the side of the waist, up and across the chest to the opposite shoulder, in a kind of an upward X pattern. Alternate hands, repeating several times.

4. ARMS. Turning the child to one side, use one of your hands to gently lift the exposed arm, holding it loosely by the wrist. Wrap your thumb and forefinger in a circle around the baby's shoulder, and draw this ring, like a tightly fitting bracelet, up along the arm toward your other hand. When you get to the wrist, switch hands. With practice, this becomes a smooth, flowing movement.

5. ARMS. Now place both hands around the arm at the child's shoulder. Move the entire hand back and forth, with the hands twisting in opposite directions away from one another, moving slowly upward toward the baby's hand, pausing at the wrist for a few more movements, then returning to the shoulder and repeating several times.

6. HANDS. Lightly grasp the child's hand, and make gentle upward strokes from the base of the palm to the base of the fingers. Massage each little finger in turn. A baby will probably grasp at your hand as you do this, but gently relax the little fingers as you work.

7. STOMACH. Placing the child on his or her back, use the flat of your hand to stroke downward, over the stomach from the base of the chest to the pelvic area, alternating hands.

8. LEGS. Now, leaving the child in the same position on his or her back, stroke the legs using the same upward movements you used for the arms. First, alternate hands with the braceletlike stroke, from the hip-end of the leg to the ankle. (Pudgy little baby thighs, with their pearly rolls of fat, probably won't fit as well as arms do in the ring formed by your thumb and forefinger, so use as much of your hand as necessary to make the movement.) Then use both hands together in the twisting/wringing stroke, moving from the thigh upward toward the foot.

9. FEET. The feet are massaged with the same strokes as the hands, first moving the thumbs up along the flat of the sole, from the heel upward to the toes. Massage each little toe, gently loosening the toes if the child curls them up. Finish with a few strokes of the flat palm of your hand along the flat sole of the child's foot.

10. BACK. Turn the baby over, so that she or he is lying face-down across your lap. Starting at the base of the back near the buttocks, slide one hand gently across the back, moving the other hand in the opposite direction. As one hand moves up, the other is moving down, all the time progressing slowly toward the baby's neck and shoulders. When you get to the top, start moving back down, and so on, back and forth several times.

11. BACK. Hold the child's buttocks with the right hand as the left hand starts at the base of the neck and strokes downward to the base of the spine. Do not put pressure on the backbone itself. After several strokes, the right hand moves down to gently grasp the child's feet, to keep the legs long and extended, and the left hand strokes from the base of the neck all the way down the legs to the ankles.

12. FACE. Finish the massage with a few gentle strokes to the face. Turn the child over again so she or he is facing up. Wipe your hands on the towel if there is any oil left on them. Rest your hands gently on the "third eye" area, above and between the eyebrows. Slowly move your fingertips outward from this center-point, along the eyebrows and past the temples, then return to center and start again.

13. FACE. Gently move your thumbs upward along the sides of the nose several times. Then rest the thumbs lightly on the child's closed eyes and move them gently down toward the corners of the mouth, moving outward to the cheeks so that the mouth is slightly stretched. Repeat the movement, from eyes to cheeks, several times.

14. ARMS. Holding the baby's hands loosely at the wrists, cross the arms across the chest, then open them outward again, like a butterfly's wings. Open and close, several times.

15. LEGS. Holding the baby's legs loosely at the feet or ankles, bring the knees to the chest, then straighten them out again. Do this up and down motion several times.

16. CHEST. Rest your hands lightly on the child's chest. Make eye contact if the child is awake, and silently express your appreciation for this child's presence in your life.

Children are a gift from the Living Mystery. The massage is done.

❧

Ashley Montagu, in his excellent book *Touching: The Human Significance of the Skin,* notes that women who are massaged during pregnancy are also more effective at giving massage to their newborns. My older children were wonderful at giving back massages during my last pregnancy, and expectant dads can also contribute. Happy moms make for happy babies, as an infant's brainwave patterns, which lay the circuitry for habitual emotional response throughout life, tend to be patterned after their mother's moods during the first year of life. Researchers at the University of

Washington found that babies of depressed mothers had significantly less brain activity in the left frontal lobe, which is the brain's center for joy and positive emotion. These early brain connections are extremely important, as they "tune" the brain to a particular pattern of response that influences subsequent brain development.

To raise loving children, be a loving parent. To raise joyful babies, be joyful. Give them lots of loving touch; talk and sing to them; stimulate their senses with beautiful sights, sounds, and aromas. Take them out into the natural world and guide them gently into making their own connection with the Earth. These are simple prescriptions from Mother Earth's healing cabinet, traditions observed by so many of our planet's ancient and aboriginal people, the effectiveness of which our science and technology is only beginning to confirm.

Aromatherapy, especially when combined with massage, is healing in ways that can be documented by science and technology as well as in ways that cannot. I personally believe that essential oils are somehow willing and able to accept the imprint of the loving intention of the person using them for healing purposes. Through the olfactory process, the essences, by virtue of their ability to gain access to the nervous system and the deepest feeling and control centers of the brain, carry this loving intention and allow it to interact at the most fundamental level of being, restoring balance, repairing or neutralizing damage, dissipating blocked energies and emotions that can adversely affect proper physiological functioning, and generally correcting the flow of love and the vital force. I believe that the use of essential oils changes people both biochemically and spiritually. Like the other plant-based remedies in this book, they are a form of love from our green relatives, extending an invitation to us and our children to reconnect with our extended family, and to come home, home to our Mother.

Dilutions

Babies
For babies over one month, use one or two drops of extremely gentle essential oils such as rose, lavender, or chamomile, in the bath or diluted in one ounce of carrier.

Children
For children from two to five years, use three to five drops of child-safe essences only diluted in one ounce of carrier.

Older Children
For older children, proportionate to body weight and taking into account skin sensitivity, use three to ten drops of essence in one ounce of carrier.

Adults
For adults, use five to twenty drops of essential oil per ounce of carrier, depending on the essence chosen and sensitivity.

Lavender and rose, because of their extreme mildness and solubility in water, are the only essential oils that are recommended for use undiluted in the bath or on the skin. All other essential oils or essential oil blends should be diluted before use in a carrier such as a cold-pressed vegetable or nut oil, milk, or a mild, unscented, natural liquid soap base.

MOTHER EARTH'S TOP TWELVE ESSENTIAL OILS

(The oils are not listed in alphabetical order, but in order of their usefulness.)

Lavender *Lavandula vera, L. officinalis*
Entire books have been written about lavender, the essential oil so beloved to those, like me, who have benefited from its many uses that it is practically synonymous with aromatherapy. The clean, refreshing beauty of its aroma has an almost universal appeal. It can be used to help alleviate practically any infection and has so many beneficial properties that scarcely a day goes by when there is not an opportunity for its use. Stress and tension, mosquito bites, burns, cuts and scrapes, fevers, and insomnia are only a few of the day-to-day conditions that can benefit from a quick application of a drop or two of lavender essence. Lavender is one of only a few essential oils that are mild enough to use undiluted on the skin, making it a handy first-aid oil to keep in the kitchen for burns, scalds, or scrapes, or to carry in a purse or pocket for sniffing in traffic jams and other stressful situations. Overall, lavender is used in aromatherapy to balance, calm, and soothe, both

physically and emotionally. Midwives have also used lavender essence for perineal repair following childbirth. A gentle sedative when used in small doses, it helps relieve spasm, harmonize the emotions, and regulate sleep patterns. A potent natural antibiotic, lavender is also an excellent essence to use in baths, massage, or diffuser blends to boost overall resistance and strengthen immune response. The aroma and exact qualities of lavender will vary somewhat, depending on where it is grown, as is the case with any natural essential oil. French lavender, for example, will generally possess more calming properties, while Spanish lavender, due to its unique chemical makeup, will tend to be more stimulating. Lavender blends beautifully with most other essential oils, except for jasmine, neroli, and sandalwood.

Rose *Rosa damascena, R. alba, R. gallica, R. centifolia*
Of the hundreds of rose species on our planet, only the four Old Rose species listed above are used for purposes of aromatherapy, in the form of steam-distilled rose essence, rose absolute, rose otto, or rose water. The chemical makeup of rose absolute and steam-distilled rose are quite different, leading chemist and researcher Dietrich Wabner to suggest that rose absolute be used in the alleviation of psychological conditions such as anxiety, depression, and insomnia, while the distilled rose oil is more effective for physical ailments such as herpes, constipation, and fungal infections. The healing properties of rose and rose water are as extensive as those of lavender, but the preciousness of rose is reflected in its price, making it costly to most families for day-to-day use. It is, however, worth the investment to have a small amount on hand for special occasions and moments of extreme stress or trauma. I refer to rose as "liquid love," and there are simply times when no other essence will do. With its age-old reputation for enhancing love on both the physical and the emotional level, rose should have a place in every home for smoothing over the conflicts and relational problems that accompany family living.

Good quality rose water contains about 1 percent of diluted rose essence and is an economical substitute that can be taken internally to strengthen the circulatory and digestive systems and to raise spirits, confidence, and assertiveness. Because of its antiseptic and skin-soothing properties, I sometimes use rose water to bathe my baby, and I also spray it lightly on the diaper area at the first sign of irritation to prevent the development of diaper rash. Rose has a particular affinity for women and their emotional and reproductive issues. A warm bath with a few drops of pure rose essence is my own personal miracle cure, transforming me from a frazzled, stressed-out workaday harridan to serene queen of home and hearth in less than twenty minutes. (Try it!) Rose is also useful in promoting parent-child bonding and averting postpartum depression. Aesthetically beautiful and possessing a broad spectrum of beneficial qualities, rose supports health and healing on all levels. It blends well with other florals, woods, spices, and precious oils, such as jasmine and neroli, and benzoin, geranium, and sandalwood.

Eucalyptus *Eucalyptus globulus, E. radiata, E. smithii, E. citriodora*
There are hundreds of varieties of eucalyptus, and the most commonly used are listed here. Eucalyptus trees are often planted in wet, swampy areas, not to drain off the water, as some believe, but to prevent the spread of malaria by preventing the breeding of the mosquitoes that carry it. Australian aborigines have been using eucalyptus for centuries or more to bind and heal wounds. The tree was first introduced to Europe in the mid-nineteenth century. Dr. Valnet's book *The Practice of Aromatherapy*[18] gives a detailed account of the powerful antiseptic and anti-infective properties of this wonderful essence, which is used in aromatherapy primarily for its effectiveness in treating respiratory conditions and preventing the spread of infection. Research has shown that eucalyptus will penetrate the lungs after it has been rubbed onto the skin. The essence can also be used alone or in conjunction with lavender, in a lukewarm bath or compress, to bring down a fever. I put my kids into a warm bath with a few drops of eucalyptus at the first sign of a cold or flu, since it helps kill germs even as they attack. Eucalyptus essence is also effective in the diffuser or in a vaporizer to alleviate coughs and congestion and disinfect the air of a sickroom. *E. citriodora* is an effective insect repellent. Eucalyptus is an excellent addition to any massage oil used for muscle aches. The essence is effective in an inhalation for sinusitis or bronchitis. Other uses include the treatment of burns and wounds, rheumatism, intestinal parasites, and migraines. Eucalyptus essential oil is also one of the few substances that can effectively remove beach tar. Blends well with bergamot, lavender, pine, and tea tree.

Tea Tree *Melaleuca alternifolia*

Entire books have been written about this exceptional essential oil. Like eucalyptus, it is also native to Australia, where Bundjalung aborigines have used it for countless centuries to treat wounds and skin problems. This essential oil was also included in World War II first-aid kits for its wound-cleansing properties, and it has actually been shown to increase in effectiveness when infection is present. A 1994 study reported by an Australian research team showed tea tree essential oil to be active against a wide variety of microbes, including *Mycobacterium smegmatis, Clostridium perfringens, Lactobacillus acidophilus, Bacteroides fragilis, Staphylococcus aureus, Serratia marcesens, Bacillus subtilis, Candida albicans,* and *Enterococcus faecalis.*[19] Tea tree oil is a powerful disinfectant and antiseptic, yet a good-quality essence is safe, nontoxic, and nonirritating. It is one of only a few natural substances that work effectively against all classes of microorganisms, from bacteria and germs to fungi. Clinical studies have proven its effectiveness against *Streptococcus,* yeast and fungal infections, cystitis, acne, and impetigo. The essence is often used in aromatherapy to combat candida or yeast conditions, athlete's foot, diaper rash, and, diluted in evening primrose oil, for herpes. Not a pretty smell, it can be used alone or blended into a powerful, multipurpose synergy with eucalyptus, lavender, and lemon.

Chamomile *Anthemis nobilis* (Roman);
Matricaria chamomilla (German)

The chamomiles are among the top essential oils overall, especially for women and children, and they share many of the same properties as lavender, although chamomile may be more costly. Still, the German, or blue, chamomile with its high azulene content, is second to none for taking the itch out of mosquito bites.

Chamomiles are used in aromatherapy for a wide variety of physical and nervous complaints, from respiratory problems to tummy aches to skin and hair care. The oil's calming effects are traditional lore. Best used in massage blends or the bath, its primary uses are as an antispasmodic and anti-inflammatory. Use chamomile in a tummy rub for nausea, colic, or digestive cramps in children, and for infantile diarrhea. Also useful for fevers brought on by overexcitement or nerves, teething, eye problems, lower backache, sensitive or dry skin, eczema, and dermatitis. Chamomile has an overall calming effect, benefiting emotional conditions such as irritability,

grief, insomnia, shock, depression, emotional blocks, and hypersensitivity. For women, chamomile can be useful to balance PMS.
Blue chamomile is particularly indicated for skin problems and
has excellent antibacterial properties, inhibiting the growth of
Staphylococcus aureus and *Haemolytic streptococcus*, which cause
scarlet fever and rheumatoid arthritis. Blends well with benzoin,
bergamot, geranium, lavender, lemon, marjoram, neroli, peppermint, rose, and ylang-ylang. For an effective headache-relieving
blend, try mixing essences of chamomile, lavender, and peppermint, and inhale the essential oil blend or dilute and rub into the
temples, headache, or forehead, where the pain is centered.

Clary Sage *Salvia sclarea*
This relative of sage is a native of southern France, Italy, and
North Africa. The herbalist John Evelyn was so taken with the
plant's healing ability that he wrote, "In short it is a plant indu'ed
with so many wonderful properties as the assiduous use of it is
said to render men immortal." Clary sage essence is generally safer
to use than sage essential oil, due to the latter's high thujone
content. Clary sage is a powerful relaxing oil, and because of the
molecule's similarity to estrogen, the oil is often used to balance
female hormonal conditions. I include it for its excellent euphoric
qualities, which in today's stressful world can be eminently useful.
Also, I have found it very useful for earaches, when diluted in
warm oil and massaged gently around the outside of the ear and
neck, which was suggested to me by the aromatherapy educator
Michael Scholes. Essence of clary sage has many properties,
including antiseptic, antispasmodic, and aphrodisiac qualities and
can be included in many blends for its general tonic effects.
Aromatherapy applications include balancing PMS and menstrual
problems, digestive cramps and colic, migraine, bronchial asthma,
muscle cramps, scalp problems, and dermatitis. Emotionally, clary
sage enhances feminine qualities, balances mood swings, and
helps alleviate tension, stress, and postnatal depression. It blends
well with lavender, tangerine, and most essential oils. Do not use
with alcohol.

Mandarin *Citrus nobilis, C. madurensis, C. reticulata var. mandarin*
Named for its popularity as a gift to Chinese noblemen, the
essence derived from the peel of the sweet fruit of the mandarin
orange has a special affinity for children, as does tangerine

(*C. reticulata*), which was hybridized from it. Although the aromas are somewhat similar, mandarin essence contains a sedative component that is not present in tangerine, and which gives the mandarin essence a superior relaxing quality. Diluted in a rich oil blend such as hazelnut and wheat germ or avocado, it is also useful for pregnant women to prevent stretch marks. Mandarin combined with neroli and sandalwood makes a beautiful-smelling relaxing blend that can be diluted in jojoba as a perfume or any cold-pressed vegetable or nut oil for a relaxing massage. A mandarin/lavender blend promotes relaxation to invite sound sleep and good dreams. Both mandarin and tangerine make excellent tummy rubs for colic in infants and young children, and for relieving nausea during pregnancy. Its sweet, sunny fragrance is popular with people of all ages, and it blends well with just about every other essence.

Helichrysum *Helichrysum angustifolium, H. italicum*
Helichrysum grows wild on the island of Corsica and is unrivaled in aromatherapy for its use on contusions, bruises, sprains, and swelling due to its marvelous anti-inflammatory properties. Because of its high ketone content, it should be used sparingly and in dilution. It is also useful in diffuser or massage blends for rhinitis, coughs, bronchitis, asthma, allergies, and arthritis. Dilute it in a blend of hazelnut oil with a little rosehip seed oil or oil of evening primrose for a skin oil that can be very effective for sensitive skin. It blends well with citruses, chamomile, and lavender or lavandin, a hybrid of lavender.

Peppermint *Mentha piperita*
Mint has been used medicinally by many ancient cultures, from the Egyptians and Chinese to the American Indians. Its use as a digestive aid goes back to ancient Greece and Rome. Peppermint essential oil is extremely concentrated and is used in aromatherapy as a strong antiseptic and anti-inflammatory. It is very effective in blends made for room sprays, diffusers, inhalations, and rubs for relieving respiratory congestion, and the essence has been shown to kill *staphylococcus* bacteria. One drop is generally plenty in a blend or bath, as it can cause sensations of intense cold or tingling. Use in a cool compress for headaches. Because of its stimulating properties, don't use peppermint before bedtime unless you really want to stay awake. It is also an

effective repellent for insects such as ants, mosquitoes, and gnats. Dilute in a sprayer bottle of water and spritz. It blends well with lavender, marjoram, orange, and tangerine.

Ravensara *Ravensara aromatica*

This aromatic essential oil from Madagascar is the aromatherapist's first choice for treating flu symptoms. It has antiseptic, antiviral, and expectorant properties and can be used as a general nerve tonic. The essence is also said to be useful for zona (shingles) and mononucleosis. In a bath, diffuser, or massage blend, it can be used alone or combined with lavender to promote sleep and help alleviate insomnia.

Cypress *Cupressus sempervirens*

Distilled from one of the oldest trees on earth, cypress was dedicated to the ancient Egyptian and Roman gods of death and the underworld. It was used medicinally by the Assyrians and by Hippocrates and has long served as a symbol of life and death. A tea made of the cones, simmered for ten minutes, is an excellent healing astringent wash for bleeding gums and hemorrhoids. The essential oil, in a 1 to 2 percent dilution in a bath oil or ointment, can be used for the same purposes. Because it aids circulation and stimulates the lymphatic system, this is another essential oil that is beneficial in improving cellulite. Cypress essential oil is also useful for controlling any excess of fluid, such as excessive perspiration or menstrual flow. A few drops on the pillow can help coughing spasms, such as those that accompany whooping cough. In a bowl or diffuser next to the bed, cypress can also be beneficial for bronchial asthma. I have also found it very effective in relieving sore throats, when swabbed on externally at the first sign of discomfort. It blends well with benzoin, bergamot, grapefruit, juniper, lavender, rosemary, and thyme.

OTHER USEFUL ESSENTIAL OILS

Benzoin *Styrax benzoin*

Not really an essential oil, benzoin is a gum resin from a tree and must be melted down. It's a nice oil to use for children because of its pleasant vanilla ice cream smell. Benzoin stimulates circulation and respiration, soothes irritated skin, and reduces nervous tension. A warming essence, it is used in aromatherapy for symptoms such as cough and sore throat that accompany colds or flu, stomach pains, and urinary tract infections. Added to your favorite lotion or cream, it makes a soothing treatment for irritated or chapped skin or chilblains. It blends well with chamomile, cypress, jasmine, lavender, lemon, myrrh, rose, or sandalwood.

Bergamot *Citrus aurantium var. bergamia*
This refreshing aromatic is popular in perfumery and is used in aromatherapy mainly for its uplifting, antidepressant, and stress-relieving properties. It is also the distinctive flavoring used in Earl Grey tea. Bergamot is an antispasmodic, useful in alleviating colic and intestinal parasites. It also stimulates the appetite. In skin care, it helps with acne, eczema, chicken pox, shingles, and cold sores. Bergamot blends well with most floral and wood oils, especially cedar, chamomile, cypress, geranium, jasmine, lavender, neroli, sandalwood, and ylang-ylang. If you are going out into the sun, do not use bergamot essential oil that has been prepared by cold expression because it contains furocoumarins, which cause sensitivity to ultraviolet light and can result in permanent pigment discoloration. Steam-distilled bergamot does not contain this chemical component and can be more safely used.

Geranium *Pelargonium roseum, P. odoratissimum*
The "poor man's rose" was once considered a powerful healer by ancient civilizations, which used it to treat cancer. Today the plant is no longer used medicinally, though the leaves are employed to scent potpourri. In aromatherapy, geranium essential oil is used for stress relief and skin care. It is helpful for women's conditions such as PMS, hormone regulation, lymphatic function, fluid retention, and congestion of the breasts while nursing. It is also used as a deodorant; for sores, burns, dry eczema, and contact dermatitis; sore throat, tonsillitis, and lice. Blend with bergamot, lemon, or citronella to create an effective insect repellent. Geranium blends well with bergamot, lavender, and rose.

Grapefruit *Citrus paradisi*
Grapefruit is another uplifting citrus essence that is useful in anti-depressant and stimulating blends. In aromatherapy it is used for PMS and cellulitis. It blends well with cypress, geranium, lavender, marjoram, and rosemary.

Jasmine *Jasminum officinale, J. grandiflorum* (absolute)
With some similar properties to rose, jasmine also has a long history in perfumery and is just as impossible to synthesize as is rose. Two thousand pounds of jasmine blossoms, handpicked in the morning the day the flowers open, make one pound of oil. Jasmine works best in sexual and reproductive problems for men and women, including lack of desire, PMS, and menstrual cramps. Jasmine is a uterine tonic, and massage with a jasmine blend in the early stages of labor can help ease pain and strengthen contractions and can also help later with expulsion of the placenta and postnatal recovery. On an emotional level, jasmine enhances confidence, relaxation, and feelings of optimism. It may also be used for voice loss. Jasmine blends well with just about every essential oil, including bergamot, black pepper, rose, and sandalwood.

Juniper *Juniperus communis*
Juniper has been used since ancient times as an antiseptic and diuretic. Only the female bush produces berries; it can take up to three years for the berries to ripen from green to frosty purple. All parts of the shrub have been used medicinally. French hospital wards once burned sprigs of juniper with rosemary for its antiseptic properties, and the essential oil is still considered an excellent household disinfectant. In aromatherapy, juniper essence is often used on an emotional/spiritual level to neutralize negative or draining energy and on a physical level as a diuretic. Blend juniper with lavender and rosemary for a good diuretic blend that can be used in bath or massage. Juniper blends well with bergamot, lavender, peppermint, and rosemary.

Lavandin *Lavandula hybrida abrialis, L.h. grosso, L.h. Reydovan, L.h. super*
This hybrid of true lavender and spike lavender has many properties in common with lavender, but without the calming or sleep-inducing effects. Because the plant yields more essential oil than true lavender, it can also be considerably less expensive.

Lemon *Citrus limonum*
One of the most vitamin-rich essential oils, lemon essence activates white corpuscles and helps combat the aging process. It is also a superior antiseptic and bactericide. It takes about three

thousand lemons to produce one kilo of lemon essential oil. Lemon oil is also useful in blends for bronchitis, colds, flu, fever, and nosebleeds. In skin care, it is used to control secretions in oily skin, to help repair broken capillaries, and to get rid of warts and corns. Because it can be irritating, like any of the citruses, use less than 1 percent in any aromatherapy blend. Two or three drops are plenty for an adult in the bathtub. It is excellent to use in room sprays and diffuser blends for general disinfecting, as it has been shown capable of neutralizing *meningococcus* and *pneumococcus* as well as diphtheritic and typhus bacillus, for time periods ranging from fifteen minutes to twelve hours. Lemon blends well with benzoin, chamomile, eucalyptus, fennel, frankincense, geranium, juniper, lavender, neroli, and ylang-ylang.

Marjoram *Origanum majorana*
Marjoram is a sleep-promoting, sedative essential oil that has analgesic, antispasmodic, and antiaphrodisiac qualities. It is used in aromatherapy to promote emotional and sexual equilibrium, to ease grief and loneliness, and to help alleviate respiratory conditions such as bronchitis, asthma, colds, and ticklish sensations in the throat and chest. It blends well with lavender.

Neroli *Citrus vulgaris, C. aurantium, C. bigardia*
This is a beautiful, fragrant essence distilled from the blossom of the bitter orange, which was used traditionally in bridal wreaths and bouquets. The essence is a good aromatherapeutic friend to the stressed-out modern woman attempting to "do it all." A drop of neroli on a cotton ball can be sniffed as a genuinely effective deep relaxant and sleep aid. Used in a massage blend, it also promotes relaxation, soothes dry, sensitive, or inflamed skin, alleviates anxiety and nervous tension and symptoms resulting from such tensions, and functions as an effective aphrodisiac. Neroli blends well with other citruses, jasmine, rose, and sandalwood.

Niaouli *Melaleuca viridiflora, M.quinquenervia viridiflora*
(a.k.a. MQV)
Once known as "gomenol," this essential oil is named for Gomen in New Caledonia, where the leaves are chewed and used in medicinal teas and the essence is used to purify water. Niaouli is closely related to cajeput, along with tea tree, another Melaleuca, but niaouli is less irritating to the skin and mucous membranes.

This essence has been used in French hospitals as an antiseptic and to protect skin from radiation burns during cobalt therapy. Laboratory tests in the 1950s found that concurrent use of niaouli increased the activity of streptomycin and penicillin, making it a good essential oil to use in conjunction with pharmaceutical antibiotics. Niaouli is used in aromatherapy as an overall disinfectant and systemic booster, and in respiratory blends. Other applications include whooping cough, sinusitis, earache, rheumatism, parasites, burns, and laryngitis. Niaouli blends well with lavender, mint, and pine.

Orange *Citrus aurantium, C. vulgaris, C. bigaridia, C. sinensis*
Native to China and India, orange trees were not used medicinally in Europe until after their importation in the seventeenth century. In aromatherapy, the uses of orange are similar to the uses of neroli, though orange does not have the sedative quality and high price tag. Like all the citruses, orange has a cheerful, antidepressant effect. It is particularly useful for improving lymphatic circulation and is also used for alleviating cellulite. Orange also helps balance the digestive system, aiding in both constipation and diarrhea. Blended with juniper and pine, it can help ease rheumatism. Orange and tangerine are wonderful oils to diffuse in the nursery. Orange blends well with many essential oils, including spice oils, lavender, and ylang-ylang.

Pine *Pinus sylvestris, P. maritimus*
Aromatic essence of pine has been in use since the eighth century, when the famous Arab physician Avicenna used it to treat pneumonia and lung infections in much the same manner it is used in aromatherapy today. Like many of the conifer oils, pine opens up the breathing passages. In Guatemala, a popular remedy for cold sufferers is to have them sleep on a bed of fresh pine boughs, which then release their volatile healing essence with every movement. Pine can also be used to promote circulation and to help alleviate kidney or liver problems, muscular and rheumatic aches, sore throat, sweaty feet, scabies, and lice. Warming, comforting, and emotionally calming, pine is an excellent oil to use in blends for overall stress relief. Pine blends especially well with eucalyptus, tea tree, and lemon.

Rosemary *Rosmarinus officinalis*

Burned as a purifying incense in ancient Greece, rosemary has been in use since antiquity for its antiseptic and antiputrefactive abilities. This stimulating essential oil is an excellent alternative to coffee, especially when one is traveling. I carry a bottle of rosemary on long trips, whether by car or plane, and inhale briefly every so often to keep me alert (always a necessity when traveling with children!). That way, especially when traveling at night, I can arrive at my destination without a case of caffeine jitters and get a good night's sleep. Rosemary essence is also used in aromatherapy for respiratory problems, muscle pains, rheumatism, arthritis, hair loss and scalp conditions, and skin problems such as sores, burns, dry skin, and acne.

Sandalwood *Santalum album*

Good-quality sandalwood, such as the mysore that is grown as a government-regulated industry in India, is hard to find, as world demand continually exceeds its availability. Sandalwood has been prized for more than two thousand years as a urinary tract disinfectant, perfume, and incense. Furniture and temples were once built of the tree's aromatic wood, the fragrance of which promotes a meditative and spiritual state of mind. It takes thirty or more years for sandalwood to reach maturity and begin producing the oil in its heartwood. The Egyptians used sandalwood in their embalming ointments, and it was used later as a cure for gonorrhea. In aromatherapy, it is used for spiritual and emotional centering, urinary tract problems, and as a general tonic for stimulating the immune system. It has also been used traditionally as an aphrodisiac and for the care of sensitive or dry skin.

Thyme *Thymus vulgaris, linalol chemotype*

The gentle linalol chemotype is a variation of thyme producing an essence that is safer and less irritating and therefore more appropriate for use with children. Thyme essential oil stimulates the production of infection-fighting white corpuscles, thereby strengthening the immune system, and it is excellent for use in blends as a preventative rub or bath during cold season. A powerful antiseptic, thyme has been shown to kill the bacteria that cause typhoid fever and dysentery as well as *Staphylococcus* and diphtheric and tuberculosis bacillus. Thyme can also be used as part of a general flushing-out and circulation-improving regimen to eliminate toxin and fluid buildup that contributes to cellulite. The red and white varieties tend to be irritating, so use sparingly or in inhalations and room sprays. Dr. Jean Valnet used to put a few drops of thyme, lavender, pine, and eucalyptus into a small burner every day to keep the air around his work area germ-free.

Ylang-ylang *Unona odaratissima, Cananga odorata*
The rich, heady aroma of this tropical "flower of flowers" is finest in the "extra super" grade. Lower grades, which are subsequent distillations after the first, are indicated by number. Ylang-ylang I is the first distillation after super, Ylang II the second, and so on. A powerful relaxant, this essence slows down breathing and rapid heartbeat and is the aromatherapist's first choice for dealing with anger and frustration-related issues, especially when they manifest as high blood pressure, heart symptoms, or urinary tract infections. Ylang-ylang is also indicated for improving sexual response, particularly in women, and for balancing the production of sebum in oily skin.

SAFETY INFORMATION

Never use an essential oil without being fully knowledgeable regarding its purity, its purpose, its safety, and its proper application. Keep essential oils stored out of the reach of children, and use only pure, aromatherapy-grade essential oils from reputable suppliers, such as those listed in the "Resource Guide" at the end of this book.

Child-Safe Essential Oils
Chamomile (Roman and German,) clary sage, dill, eucalyptus, geranium, jasmine, lavender, lemon, mandarin, neroli, niaouli, orange, peppermint, pine, rose, rosemary verbenon, tangerine, tea tree, thyme linalol, ylang-ylang

Toxic Essential Oils
(Do not use for aromatherapy)
Ajowan, bitter almond, boldo, buchu, calamus, camphor, cornmint, horseradish, mugwort, mustard, pennyroyal, rue, sassafras, savin, savory, tansy, thuja, wintergreen, wormseed, wormwood

Essential Oils to Avoid During Pregnancy
I believe that all essential oils should be avoided during the first trimester. Thereafter, a qualified medical practitioner should be consulted regarding the use of essential oils during pregnancy. Aromatherapy can be very useful during labor, delivery, and post-partum. Midwives often can give advice in this regard. Generally, avoid any of the toxic essential oils listed above, as well as basil, bay laurel, birch, clove, marjoram, myrrh, origanum, tarragon, and thyme.

Irritating Essential Oils
(Not to be used in bath or massage blends)
Cassia, cinnamon, clove, origanum

Potential Irritants
(Discontinue use if irritation occurs)
Bay laurel, benzoin, citronella, costus, geranium (Reunion), ginger, litsea cubeba, peppermint, Peru balsam, pine, spearmint, terebinth, thyme, ylang-ylang

Phototoxic Essential Oils
(Do not use before or during exposure to the sun)
Angelica, bergamot (cold pressed), bitter orange, cumin, lemon, lime, opoponax, verbena

CHAPTER SIX

NATURE GAMES, CRAFTS, and ACTIVITIES

There was a child went forth every day,
*   and the first object he looked upon,*
*   that object he became,*
And that object became part of him for the day
*   or a certain part of the day,*
Or for many years or stretching cycles of years.
The early lilacs became part of this child,
And grass and white and red morning glories,
*   and white and red clover, and the son of the phoebe-bird,*
And the third-month lambs and the sow's pink-faint litter,
*   and the mare's foal, and the cow's calf.*

—Walt Whitman (1819–1892)

I f your child was the one described in Whitman's poem, what are the objects he or she would be assimilating each day? A daily visual and experiential diet of video games, plastic toys, pavement, automobiles, and fast-food restaurants will produce a human being very different from the one described above. For those who dwell in urban or suburban environments, a connection with Mother Earth must be deliberately sought out and cultivated. For most children, this will not happen by itself. Children are not always aware of their choices, or how they're being influenced and conditioned by the choices being made for them by adult caretakers and their daily environment. A fourth-grader quoted in *Sierra* magazine said, "I like to play indoors better 'cause that's where all the electrical outlets are." This is a child who has never experienced the beauty and magic of nature.

The sights, sounds, smells, tastes, and experiences of childhood have very real developmental implications. Children who have been conditioned to equate "strawberry" with an artificial flavor, such as that used in Kool-Aid or Jell-O products, cannot identify the taste or smell of the natural berry as "strawberry." For those born before 1972, when most of us still spent most of our free time playing outside, the fondest olfactory memories of childhood were natural in origin, such as fruit or flower aromas, spices, or baking bread. Those born after the 1970s tend to wax nostalgic about artificial fragrances, such as those used in Play Dough or crayons. What effect this actually has on a child's developing worldview has not yet been analyzed, but I hardly think it can contribute to a greater sense of oneness and connection with nature. What are we teaching our children to respond to and love?

Experience is the best teacher, emotion tethers memory, and repetition cements the neural connections that lead from the great halls of learning to the innermost sanctums of wisdom and mastery. The games and activities in this chapter are open-ended, experiential in nature. Approach them with a sense of play. Rachel Carson, who chilled the world with her warning of the long-term effects of pesticide use in her classic book *Silent Spring,* spent her last years, as she was dying of cancer, lovingly sharing nature with her grandnephew Roger. She recorded these experiences in her last book, *The Sense of Wonder,* in which she observed, "The sharing includes nature in storm as well as calm, by night as well as day, and is based on having fun together rather than on teaching. I sincerely believe that for the child, and for the parent seeking to guide him, it is not half so important to know as to feel." So keep your ears and eyes, mind, heart, and spirit open as you and your child engage in these activities.

NATURE GAMES

Those who contemplate the beauty of the earth find reserves of strength that will endure as long as life lasts. There is something infinitely healing in the repeated refrains of nature the assurance that dawn comes after night, and spring after the winter.

—Rachel Carson, *The Sense of Wonder*

Spirit Hunter: This is a silent nature awareness and at-one-ment exercise that was once used to develop hunting skills among American Indians. It is better suited to an older child, since it works best if the child can be left alone. The best place to try this is in an area where there is both a short- and long-range view of earth and sky, although it can be performed anywhere. Sitting very quietly and very still, the child is instructed to blend in with the natural surroundings. Everything has a spirit. The grasses and trees, the birds, the insects, even the rocks have their own particular energy and way of being. If she or he sits in an open and receptive state, soon something will intuitively call for attention. It may be a bird, a plant or flower, or an animal. That which is calling has a message, something important to say. What is it trying to communicate? This form of hunting is not an aggressive pursuit of another creature for the purpose of ending its life, but a quiet search for connection with another living thing. When in a connected state in nature, amazing things can happen. Animals may approach closely instead of running away. There is also the wonderful and comforting realization that we are always surrounded by other forms of life with whom we can make friends. A human being who is capable of forming relationships not only with other people but with all of Mother Earth's children will never be lonely or alone.

Who Am I? Pictures or names of animals are pinned to the backs of participants, and children must gather clues as to their animal's identity by asking for information from other players. This is a wonderful game for children of all ages, and a great ice breaker at a party or gathering. We played it for the first time in a children's program of activities at a Wisconsin state park. To make animal placards that can be used more than once, use cardboard or stiff paper, about 8 x 10 inches works fine, and punch holes in the two upper corners, then tie through a piece of string so it can hang comfortably around a child's neck. For children who can't read, pictures of animals can be drawn or pasted on. Older children can get by with just the names, written in large type. There should be one animal paper or placard for each child. The placard is hung around the child's neck, facing outward so the child can't see what animal he or she is. The children then show each other the animal on their backs and ask each other for clues. "Do I have four legs?" "Do I have feathers?" "Do I eat meat?" They must ask for one clue from each child present before they can ask a second question of the same person, but they are not allowed to guess what they are. When they think they know what animal they are, they sit down in a designated area until all the children have gathered there. One at a time they stand up and repeat what they have learned about themselves, then they announce their conclusion as to what they are, which may be correct or sometimes hilariously wrong.

Food Chain: We played this game as part of an enrichment unit in Earth Awareness that I taught for my son's second grade. First we cut strips of construction paper, about 1 x 3 inches in size, large enough to be glued or taped into a chain-type link. Blue paper links represented water, green represented plants, and the various other colors were for animals (including humans), fish, birds, and insects. Then we wrote on each strip of paper what it stood for, and put them in a pile. Players draw one or more (depending on the size of the group) strips of paper, then mix and match between themselves as they figure out who is connected to what. For instance, a blue link for water could be connected to almost any other link, since all living things require food. A brown link representing an insect could be attached to a plant, which it eats, at one end, and a bird, which eats it, at another. In the second-grade class, I drew a black dot on some of the links, indicating the presence of pesticides or poisons, which made visually clear how such things move through the environment and into the food chain. When all the links were put together, we connected them to a big yellow cutout of the sun, on which almost all life on our planet depends.

Moon Chart: This was an assignment from a creative teacher at my children's elementary school. Give the children calendars and have them go outside and look at the moon each night through the course of one lunar cycle. Each night they must then draw a picture of what they see as the moon moves through its various stages. Some nights the moon will be obscured by clouds or rain. Some nights the moon will rise very late. If you live in a place where they can sit outside to observe, have them also record any thoughts or observations.

Mini-World Census: Who Lives Here? Perhaps because they feel so much smaller than the adult world surrounding them, children are fascinated with tiny things. In this activity, a magnifying glass can be very useful. Mark off a small plot of earth with string, which can be wrapped around the stems of four fairly sturdy plants growing there. If there are no plants strong enough, put slender sticks into the ground and wrap the string around them. The plot should be no bigger than twelve inches by twelve inches. The children are going to take a census for Mother Earth. Older children can make a count and record it on a small clipboard hung from a string around their necks, that can make them feel more like an "official" census taker. Who lives in this tiny plot of land and where? How many are there? Who is just passing through? What can the children see, hear, touch, or smell to tell them more about how these little creatures live?

Scavenger Hunt: This is a natural variation on the classic party game. First, check out the area in which the game is to be played and include items that will lead the child into contact with whatever mysteries and delights it has to offer. Beyond just a list of objects to find, such as leaves, stones, or seeds, you can also include descriptions that will encourage a child to think creatively, for example, "Something an ant might find delicious," "Something a bird could use to build a nest," or "Something a fairy could use as a hat." Give a time limit, and when the time is up, have the players come back and share their results. If you play this as a party game and include prizes, be sure to have a reward on hand for everyone who participates. In deepening our friendship with Mother Earth, everybody wins.

No Car/No Electricity Days: This activity is best for weekends and requires some planning ahead of time. No Electricity Days can be difficult to execute completely. (I had to leave my refrigerator running.) But a lot can be learned from not flipping on a light switch, television, or appliance for twenty-four hours. Along with enhancing their awareness of how we use electricity, and consciously giving a break to those resources being used to create electricity, my kids really enjoyed those quiet, candlelit evenings without the habitual distractions that divert us from simply being with and experiencing each other. Also, on No Car Days we found ourselves pleasantly surprised by how it felt to slow down, to abandon our usual frenetic schedule of driving from this activity to that. Instead we found ourselves walking around our neighborhood, enjoying the sights, sounds, and people we had become too busy to notice.

Blindfolded Nature Walks

Being blindfolded encourages us to move away from our culturally dominant visual sense to experience and relate to nature more fully with our less-called-upon senses of hearing, touch, and smell. There are several ways to set up this type of exercise.

Hand-on-the-Shoulder-in-Front Variation: Map out a ten- to fifteen-minute walk in advance, which leads through various types of terrain, in and out of sunlight and shadows, past some aromatic bushes or plants if possible, through or alongside running water such as a stream or brook. The leader is not blindfolded and sets up those following in a line, in which each participant keeps a hand on the shoulder of the person in front of him or her for guidance. Six people is the maximum workable number. The walk is conducted in silence. When it's over, take the participants aside before the blindfolds are removed. Then ask them to work together to recreate the route they just walked.

Rope Guide Variation: Especially effective with young children, this version is set up with a shorter walk, using a rope tied along the whole route as a guide. Each blindfolded participant has a seeing guide who walks alongside him or her. The blindfolded player holds onto the rope, with the guide being present only to ensure safety. Flags can be tied to the rope at certain points to indicate something special that can be touched or experienced, such as a fern, a rock, or a flowering bush.

Tree Variation: After being blindfolded, each participant is led to a tree that she or he is instructed to explore as fully as possible. Encourage the child to put his or her arms around the tree to feel how big it is, to experience the texture of the bark and any smell it may have. Can s/he hear the song of any birds that might have a nest or be visiting here? After exploring the tree, hands, ears, and noses can also be used to discern what may be located nearby, such as rocks, stones, or plants, and what is on the ground at the base of the trunk. After ten minutes or so, the participants are led a short distance away and their blindfolds are removed. Can they go back now and find their trees?

Nighttime Variation: Of all the blindfold games my children and I have played, this is my all-time favorite. I experienced this version at a family nature camp hosted by Earth Skills in the mountains of southern California. Because it is played at night and involves a fair amount of uncertainty, it is generally not appropriate for very young children. After being blindfolded, participants are taken on a short walk through various kinds of terrain, using the hand-to-shoulder method described above. One by one, each player is silently taken aside and left alone at a certain point along the trail and instructed to wait for the sound of the drum. The leader chooses a point equidistant from the players, preferably in an area without dangerous obstacles. The blindfolded participants must then find their way to the leader by listening to the beat of the drum, sensing and moving around any obstacles such as trees, bushes, or rocks that may be in their path. Depending on how far and through what terrain the players have to journey in the dark, it can be fascinating, frightening, frustrating, and a whole lot of fun. I love this game because, on a feeling level, it's just like life.

NATURE CRAFTS

In the end, we will conserve only what we love, we will love only what we understand, we will understand only what we are taught.

—Baba Dioum

Nature crafts celebrate the beauty and diversity of our planet in a hands-on way that teaches both aesthetic appreciation and respect. Southwestern Indian tribes believed that things such as baskets, lovingly handcrafted of natural materials, had a spirit of their own. A basket was not only an object for practical use; it was respected and appreciated as a valuable and contributing member of the family. Making items for household use also keeps us in touch with the reality that everything we use comes from Mother Earth, either directly or indirectly. All of us need to be reminded from time to time that the things we use don't just come from "the store."

Preserved Flowers: Flowers can be preserved by several methods and then used for decorative purposes on stationery, candles, or in dried arrangements. The blossoms can be pressed by putting them between two pieces of plain or waxed paper, which are then slipped into the pages of a heavy book and left to dry for several weeks. Flowers that are too big or fleshy to press can be preserved with sand or glycerin. Using the sand method, a layer of clean sand (such as is available at toy or gardening supply stores) is sprinkled into the bottom of a box or pan. The flowers are placed blossom side down in the sand, and more sand is sprinkled over the blooms until they are covered. Let sit in a warm, dry place for several weeks until the flower has dried. Or mix a half cup of glycerin with one cup of water and heat it almost to the boiling point. Pour the glycerin into a tall container and place the flower inside it, stem side down, as if placing a bouquet in water. Put it in a dark place until it starts to darken, then hang it upside down in a dry, warm room out of sunlight.

Recycled Herb Paper: Recycle your old newsprint or computer paper and transform it into something beautiful to enhance your home or give as a gift. Shred the paper in a shredder, or cut it into small pieces. Soak the shredded paper in warm water overnight. Using a blender, briefly puree ¼ cup soaked paper with about three cups of water. Add ¼ teaspoon laundry starch that has been diluted in a little water. Fill a big plastic bowl with the paper pulp. You will also need two frames the size of the paper you want to create (8½" x 11" is standard letter size). Sturdy, inexpensive wooden picture frames serve nicely. Staple netting tightly to one frame. The other frame is left empty. Hold the frames together and dip them vertically into the bowl full of pulp. Lay the frames down flat, empty frame up, under the surface of the water, then slowly raise it out, still holding it flat. When you've set it down, lift off the empty frame. Pressed flowers, leaves, or herbs, even small seeds can be placed on top of the paper pulp and left to dry into the sheet. When the paper is dry, loosen and remove it from the frame. To scent herbal paper, store the dried sheets in a tightly closed box or tin with bunches of lavender or rosemary, herbal sachets, or cotton balls to which you've added essential oils of your choice. Let it sit in the box or tin for about a month to fully absorb the scent. The homemade paper can then be decoratively boxed as stationery or placed in the bottoms of drawers to scent clothing or linen.

Beeswax Candles: Beeswax candles can be made either with melted blocks of beeswax or by rolling "foundation," which consists of beeswax sheets embossed with a honeycomb pattern. "Foundations" are used by beekeepers to encourage bees to build their combs in the wooden frames that line man-made hives. Block beeswax can be purchased from hobby shops or beekeepers. Melt beeswax in a double boiler, which can be created by suspending a coffee can or stainless steel bowl above a pot of boiling water. (Do not use metal other than stainless steel, as it may discolor the beeswax.) Ordinary twine or string can be dipped into the molten wax, then hung up to harden in a straight line. Molds can be purchased from a hobby shop, but they tend to be expensive. For home use, little, bathroom-size Dixie paper cups make excellent (and cheap!) molds for votive-size candles. Simply pour the melted beeswax into the cups. Then, as the wax begins to cool and congeal, poke in a length of the dipped string as a wick. Let the candles cool overnight and peel off the paper cup. Pure beeswax is beautiful as is and doesn't require color chips or hardener. Pressed flowers can be used to decorate the sides of the candle. Use a paintbrush to paint on melted beeswax as glue to hold flowers in place. Or, holding the candle by the wick, dip it in hot water for a few seconds, then roll it in dried herbs, pressing them into the softened outer layer of wax. For scented candles, simply add a handful of aromatic herbs such as rosemary, lavender, or lemon verbena to the melted wax. Strain the wax before pouring it into molds.

Herbal Toy Dough: Mix 2 cups of white flour with 1 cup of salt and 1 cup of strong herbal infusion or tea. Knead until soft and smooth. Roll out on wax paper and cut into shapes with cookie cutters. Add a loop on the front where a sprig of herb can be tucked. To make hanging or Christmas ornaments, poke a hole near the top with a toothpick for threading a hanger or ribbon. Bake at 300 degrees F for one hour. Allow to cool, then paint or varnish.

Potpourri Ornaments: Insert a long thin stick or wire into a small Styrofoam ball, such as can be found at craft stores. Hold the stick or wire as you roll the ball in glue until the surface of the ball is completely covered. Then roll the ball in dried aromatic herbs such as lavender, rosemary, rose and calendula petals, and tiny bits of citrus peel. Tie a ribbon around it as a hanger, fastening it in place with a pin pushed into the ball. Essential oils can be dropped onto the ornament's surface to intensify or freshen the scent.

Creams and Lotions: Any leftover beeswax can be saved to make natural creams and lotions. Other ingredients include a kind of cold-pressed oil, or infused herbal oil, floral water or hydrolate, and essential oils. Heat 1 cup of nut or vegetable oil in a double boiler. (I have used a Pyrex bowl resting in a saucepan.) Melt in a small chunk (about the size of the business end of a spoon) of beeswax. The more beeswax you use, the thicker and harder the finished cream will be. Remove the mixture from heat, and whisk or beat in about $1/2$ cup of home-distilled lavender water (or other floral water). Continue to beat until the mixture is just warm, adding 10 to 15 drops of the essential oils of your choice. Then pour the finished product into a small glass or plastic jar and allow it to cool completely before closing the top. This mixture will keep for about two or three weeks. For maximum shelf life, use a clean stick or spoon instead of your fingers to remove the cream, or put lotion into a pump-top container to prevent bacterial contamination.

Stuffed Sleepers: I keep my old silk skirts and shirts and turn them into sleepytime pillows. The shape can be a simple square or rectangle sewn on three sides, then turned inside out and filled with soothing, sleep-inducing herbs such as dried lavender or chamomile flowers, rose petals, or hops. Finish sewing by hand. Make a little pillowcase to fit over the pillow, which can then be removed and washed as necessary. Sleepytime bunnies or bears can be made by the same method. Just make a pattern in the shape of your child's favorite animal, sew around it except for a small opening, turn it right side out, stuff with herbs, and sew closed. A few drops of essential oil can be added to intensify the aroma.

Apple Annie: Peel an apple, then carve a face into it. Soak overnight in salt water (1 tablespoon of salt dissolved in 2 cups of warm water). Weight the apple to keep it down in the water if necessary. The next day, mount it on a stick or dowel with a stand-up base. Push cloves in for eyes, and dress her up in scraps of brightly colored cloth. As she dries, Apple Annie's face wrinkles up. Kids find this highly entertaining, though moms may react with a slight inexplicable depression. This can be a great way to get in touch with your own mortality, especially if you haven't had your midlife crisis yet.

Homemade Wrapping Paper: Cut a potato in half, then carve a simple stencil design into the potato. Dip the potato "stamp" into brightly colored tempera paint, then stamp the color onto freezer paper in repetitive patterns.

Herbal Aroma Beads: Mix 3 tablespoons powdered orris root, 2 tablespoons powdered benzoin, 1 tablespoon ground cinnamon, 1 tablespoon ground nutmeg or mace, 1 teaspoon ground cloves. Dissolve 1 teaspoon gum tragacanth into 3 tablespoons rose water, then mix with the spices to form a paste. Roll the mixture into beads, then pierce the wet beads with a needle and string on heavy thread to dry. (The ingredients I mention can generally be found wherever bulk herbs are sold. See "Resource Guide.")

Lavender Hangers: Keep clothes moth-free and smelling fresh with lavender hangers. Using a wooden strip hanger or form, bind bunches of dried lavender stalks against the hanger by winding strips of unbleached muslin. Cover the hanger with a brightly patterned fabric sleeve. Squeeze to freshen the fragrance, or sprinkle on a few drops of lavender essential oil. Or hang little muslin drawstring bags filled with dried lavender flowers from your regular hangers to get the same moth-repellent, scented effects. These can also be put under the cushions of your sofa or chairs, to release a sweet aroma whenever someone sits down.

CHAPTER SEVEN

BATH TIME

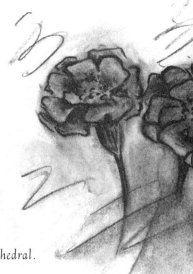

Thy baths shall be the juice of July flowers,
Spirit of roses and of violets . . .

—Ben Jonson (1572–1637)

I have had a good many more uplifting thoughts,
creative and expansive, . . . in well-equipped
American bathrooms than I have ever had in any cathedral.

—Edmund Wilson (1895–1972)

ince the dawn of human history, water has been used for physical, emotional, and spiritual cleansing. Like the developing fetus floating in a warm sea of amniotic fluid, life on Earth first evolved in water, giving us an ancestral link to this all-important fluid. Even now, our bodies still contain about 60 percent water. Soaking in a warm tub redolent with herbs, salts, or fragrant essences soothes away tensions and can be deeply comforting, reminding us of an earlier, prenatal state of oneness and our primordial beginnings.

For working parents who don't see their children all day long, bath time can be an important time for play, fun, and bonding. The healing stories included in the next chapter can be read at bath time as well as at bedtime. My kids love it when I read to them in the bath.

A BRIEF HISTORY OF THE BATH

The first known bathroom was installed almost four thousand years ago in the palace of King Minos on the island of Crete, although there is evidence that there may have been earlier versions in India and Babylon five or six thousand years ago. The Cretan king's bath was designed by the architectural genius Daedalus, also known for creating the labyrinth that housed the Minotaur and creating the mythical wings of his son Icarus, who flew too close to the sun. A terra-cotta bathtub in the palace is believed to have belonged to the queen. Bathwater was carried in by hand but was carried away by an early plumbing system of terra-cotta drains.

Ancient Egyptians were taking showers three thousand years ago, and they had bathrooms in their palaces at the time of the Exodus. Scented oils of sesame, almond, castor, and olive as well as rendered camel fat were used for bath and body, blended according to sacred, secret formulas by priests in the temples. Antony and Cleopatra had no need for soap, using a kind of abrasive scrub made with fragrant oils and white sand instead. Several hours a day were devoted to bathing by the upper class, who employed slaves to heat the water, lay out the towels, and massage and anoint them.

Around 1500 B.C., bathrooms also appeared in the Fertile Crescent of Mesopotamia. Some of the pipes, sewers, and toilets installed then still work today. Soap plant grew in this area, and it was used for cleansing the body.

The ancient Greeks offered a bath, followed by an anointing with fragrant natural perfumes, to welcome weary travelers. They bathed in birdbath-shaped marble tubs and also used showers and steam baths. Public baths, appended to their gymnasia, had only cold water to perk up the athletes before a sport, since hot baths were considered effeminate. The women of Greece were required by law to be well groomed, and could be fined for looking unkempt in public. Galen, a Greek physician of the second century, suggested washing with soap for medicinal purposes.

It was the hedonistic Romans, however, who fully developed the art of bathing. They started inauspiciously enough, the grubby early Romans splashing off dirt in the Tiber River once every nine days or so, before they went to market. Within five centuries they had developed an elaborate system of pipes and aqueducts. In 21 B.C., Agrippa built the first public bath. The groundwork was now laid, and by the time of Augustus, bathing became a Roman passion. The construction of bathhouses was subsidized by the government. Artists and architects created magnificent mosaics, gilded and vaulted ceilings, tiled walkways, marble columns, tubs, and arches, statues, vases, and bas-reliefs. The entire population of present-day Windsor, Connecticut, or Yuba City, California, could have bathed at the same time in the magnificent Caracalla public baths, which had a capacity of about eighteen thousand. During the fourth century, when the Roman Empire was at its apogee, the city of Rome contained 11 public baths, 1,352 public fountains and cisterns, and 856 private baths. Three hundred gallons of water were provided for each Roman citizen to use every day, about twice as much as is used by the average American.

Beyond mere cleanliness, Roman baths also provided social and cultural activities, housing conference rooms, libraries, theaters, art galleries, temples, and exercise rooms. Typically they were open from early afternoon until dark. In the baths, upper and lower classes mixed freely. At one o'clock, when the water was heated, a bell would ring, and the bathing day was begun. After paying the admission fee, the Roman bather went to the *apodyterium,* where he was helped to undress, then into the *unctuarium,* a heated massage room, for a full-body rubdown with oil. Then it was off to the *spaeristerium,* to exercise and raise a sweat. In the *calidarium,* a steam or hot bath cleansed away impurities, which were removed with metal scrapers called strigils. Next came another massage, followed by a cleansing water bath. Then a quick, tepid rinse in the *tepidarium* preceded a cold bath in the *frigidarium.* Back at the *unctuarium,* the Roman bather received a manicure and a final aromatic massage, emerging five hours later, feeling like a million quadrans and smelling like a rose, Rome's official flower.

Those who were wealthy enough to have a bath in the home spared no expense in appointing the room with marble tubs and silver pipes and faucets. Some had swing tubs, suspended from the ceiling by ropes. As in Egypt, slaves prepared the bath, which often contained rose water or rose-scented oils or unguents. Poppea, Nero's indulgent wife, bathed in asses' milk or a tubful of mashed strawberries. Even the soldiers of the great Roman armies were partial to bathing, carrying portable copper bathtubs with them on all their forays.

When Rome was conquered and the empire collapsed, bathing fell out of fashion for hundreds of years, having acquired a poor reputation through association with Roman decadence and decay. Eighth-century monks bathed in wooden tubs, once a week on Thursdays by papal decree, while the general population of the godly were permitted a quick cleanup on Sunday before attending religious services.

In the twelfth century, the returning Crusaders brought the concept of bathing back to Europe from Arabia. The Turkish hammam was a similar, though simpler version of the Roman bath, containing a series of warm, hot, and steam rooms and a small tub of cold water. The Crusaders christened them "stews" and, on their return from the East, intrigued their hydrophobic peers with their newly acquired habits of floating rose petals on their bathwater and sprinkling themselves *après-bains* with rose water. By the late Middle Ages, communal bathing had become a respectable social pastime for the European upper class, although the Church continued to frown upon the mixing of the sexes. Dinner and engagement parties were held in large bathtubs, with the ladies displaying their finery from the water line up. By the fourteenth and fifteenth centuries, public baths were once again popular meeting places, where everyone, from nuns and monks to young women and old men, got clean and naked together, or watched from the galleries as others did so. Floating food and gambling tables provided entertainment, and eventually some of the baths set aside small rooms for prostitution. The Italian words *bordello* and *bagnio,* which originally referred to the Turkish-style public baths, took on their tarnished meanings as a result.

When the Spaniards stumbled upon the civilizations of South America, they were scandalized by the elaborate bathing and aromatic massage indulged in by the Aztecs who, like most highly developed civilizations, devoted many pleasurable hours in pursuit of cleanliness.

Anne Boleyn angered her husband King Henry VIII of England by allowing men to fill their glasses and toast her with her bathwater. Anne and Henry's daughter, Queen Elizabeth, had a bathtub but rarely used it. Her cousin, Mary, Queen of Scots, had the married women of her court bathe in wine, while the maidens soaked in milk. During this time, soap was used mainly for laundry, or by the very rich, while general cleansing was done with toilet and floral waters brewed in home stills.

Madame Pompadour, mistress of the French king Louis XIV, bathed in an octagonal tub made of pink marble, ten feet wide and three feet deep, which was given to her by the king. Napoleon, who liked hot baths, also gave a bathtub to Josephine. The emperor's sister Pauline bathed in milk, whereas Wellington preferred cold water. In Paris in the eighteenth century, two tubs were used, one for washing, one for bathing, as in the Japanese tradition.

While American Indians bathed using natural cleansers such as soapwort, yucca, or agave, the early colonists thought bathing was bad for the health and made bathing illegal in several states. Benjamin Franklin was one of the few exceptions, having gotten in the habit of bathing while in Europe. But had he tried to take a bath more than once a month in Philadelphia, he could have been arrested and sent to jail. There were laws in early America regulating the sale and purchase of bathtubs. Even the White House had no fixed bathtub until 1851, when President Millard Fillmore had one installed.

The first public bath in America opened in New York in 1852. By 1895 the state required free public baths in all cities of fifty thousand people or more. For a nickel you could rent a towel and bar of soap to go along with it. In those days, soap was usually made at home in big batches, a year's worth at one time, from saved-up fat drippings and wood ash mixed with lye. Bar soap, individually wrapped, as we know it, wasn't available in the United States until after 1830. Ivory Soap, the first floating bar, was introduced by Proctor and Gamble in 1878 as "White Soap." Four years later the company added the marketing slogan "99 $^{44}/_{100}$% pure," thereby kicking off the multibillion-dollar toiletries and cosmetics industry of today. Lest you think that advertising gobbledygook is a recent invention, read this 1932 Procter and Gamble blurb about its famous soap: "Its origin was strictly mathematical and precise. It is the result of an analysis made generations ago by a chemist of national fame and was corroborated by an equally celebrated authority. As for the meaning of 'pure' the statement means that Ivory Soap as far as it is possible analytically to determine by chemical analysis, is 99 $^{44}/_{100}$% pure."

In nineteenth-century America, it was possible to take a shower, but it required a fair amount of work to pump the water up to the shower spout. The Virgina Stool Shower solved the problem by creating a shower with a built-in bicycle-style pump. As long as you kept pedaling, the shower kept on spraying.

The first private bath in an American home was a richly appointed, luxurious bathing oasis installed by wealthy George Vanderbilt in 1855. Rich people in general quickly joined in the bathroom-building fad, although they still only used the bath on

Saturday nights. Then Thomas Crapper invented the flushing toilet in 1872, and the bathroom was transformed, literally, from the room around the bathtub into the tiled toilet, sink, and tub chamber most of us recognize today.

Bathing for Health

At different times in history, baths have been prescribed medicinally and for their overall health benefits. A hot bath, with massage, can bring blessed relief to overworked, tense, or tired muscles. A bath that is higher in temperature than body heat is considered a hot bath, but a bath should not exceed 110 degrees F. Hot baths should be taken for no longer than twenty minutes and should be avoided altogether by those who are more than ten pounds overweight, have heart problems or high blood pressure, and have dry or sensitive skin. Hot baths are also not appropriate for infants or small children.

Follow a hot bath with a cool (not cold) rinse, or a friction rub using a natural alcohol-based cologne splash or witch hazel to help normalize body temperature. Witch hazel extract can also be used as a scalp rub to invigorate the scalp and alleviate dandruff. It also has astringent and anti-inflammatory properties that make it useful as a skin wash to soothe burns, scrapes, bites, or itchy skin. Witch hazel can be used alone or combined half and half with rose water, a few drops of glycerin, and/or essential oils to make an excellent facial toner.

Herbed vinegar infusions, aromatic oils, or aromatherapy bath salts can enhance the relaxation sought from a hot bath and can be used in warm or cool baths as well. Oils and salts can be blended, or essential oils dropped in, just before getting into the tub. Herbal infusions and infused oils need to be prepared further in advance.

Bath Vinegars

Dried Herb Method: Slowly heat two and a half cups of vinegar (white, red wine, or apple cider are all good choices), to which you've added a handful of dried herbs, to a boil, then turn off the heat and allow the mixture to infuse overnight. In the morning, strain the liquid and pour it into a bottle, then refrigerate. It should last quite a long time. However, if it looks cloudy, toss it.

Fresh Herb Method: Fresh herb vinegars can also be made by loosely filling a bottle with fresh herbs, then filling the bottle with vinegar. Let the bottle sit in a sunny spot for two weeks, then strain out the herb.

Muscle-Soothing Bath Herbs: Borage, comfrey, English mallow, eucalyptus, ginger, juniper berries, lavender, mustard (powder)

Healing Bath Herbs: Calendula flowers, comfrey, nettle, plantain, spearmint, yarrow

Relaxing Bath Herbs: Chamomile, hops, jasmine flowers, lavender, lemon balm, linden flowers, rose petals, valerian, vervain

Stimulating Bath Herbs: Basil, bay leaves, eucalyptus, fennel, mint, pine, rosemary, sage, thyme

Quick Bath Vinegar: Add 10 to 20 drops (for an adult, no hot baths for kids!) of essential oils of your choice to 4 cups of room-temperature vinegar and shake well. This makes enough for two baths.

Bath Salts
Mix 1/2 cup sea salt, 1/2 cup baking soda, and 1/2 cup Epsom salts in a bowl. Add 10 to 20 drops of essential oils of your choice and mix well. This makes enough for two baths.

Sea of Milk and Honey Bath
Boil 1 1/2 cups water, pour it into a mixing bowl, and stir in 1 cup honey until dissolved. Add 1 cup whole milk. After dissolving bath salts in the bathwater, add the milk and honey mixture.

Bath and Body Oils
Hot baths can dry the skin, a condition that can be alleviated by adding oil to the bath or rubbing a small amount of oil into the skin after getting out of the water, before toweling off. Dried herbs can be infused in any cold-pressed nut or vegetable oil, using about 1 pound of herbs fully immersed in 1 gallon of oil. Strain through cheesecloth and allow the oil to drip through. A quicker method is simply to add essential oils to a carrier oil at a dilution of about 1 to 2 percent. For instance, to 1 ounce of oil, add 5 to

10 drops of essences. Then add about a tablespoon of this blended oil to the bath just before you get in, mixing it with your hand. Bath and body oils can be used in conjunction with warm baths, too.

Muscle-soothing Essential Oils: Blue chamomile, cypress, eucalyptus, grapefruit, juniper, lavender, marjoram, rosemary, tea tree, thyme

Healing Essential Oils: Chamomile, eucalyptus, lavender, rose, tea tree, thyme

Relaxing Essential Oils: Chamomile, clary sage, lavender, mandarin, marjoram, neroli, rose, sandalwood, ylang-ylang

Stimulating Essential Oils: Bergamot, cypress, geranium, grapefruit, lemon, peppermint, rosemary

ॐ

Warm baths are those most frequently indulged in, for their relaxing, soothing, stress-relieving, and sleep-promoting effects. Body temperature, or just slightly above, is ideal for a warm bath. According to Beverly Frazier, coauthor of *The Bath Book,* you can increase elimination of toxins by drinking small quantities of cold water while in a warm bath, which stimulates kidney function.

Bath enhancements such as salts, oils, and vinegars are also wonderful with a warm bath. Milk baths soften the skin. Oatmeal baths are skin-soothing and therapeutic and especially useful for skin conditions and ailments such as chicken pox. When my children had chicken pox, the combination of twice-daily oatmeal baths, essential oils, and plenty of pumpkin pie (rich in beta carotene) helped them come through all that itchy misery with their skin beautifully intact.

Bath Bags
To minimize cleanup and keep little bits of dried or fresh herbs from sticking to you or your kids when you get out of the tub, bath bags can't be beat. You can buy or sew little bags from cheesecloth or gauze to fill with bath goodies, and even decorate them and tie them with a ribbon to give as gifts. If aesthetics don't

matter, the foot end of an old nylon or pair of pantyhose can be cut off, stuffed, and tied shut with a rubber band or bit of string. In a pinch, you can also use a clean handkerchief or a lightweight washcloth. Just spread it open, pile the ingredients in the middle, bring the corners together and tie with string. Toss the bag into a warm bath, or hang it from the faucet as the tub fills. Once you're in the bath, you can use the bath bag as a scrubber to buff and smooth your skin to a silken texture, especially if you add a little cornmeal or ground almond to your bath bag blend. When you're done with it, dump the remnants into your garden or compost pile, and wash the cloth.

Soothing and Invigorating Baths

Chamomile Cream Bath: This soothing bath softens skin and melts away nervous tension. It can be made with dry or fresh ingredients. Dry Method: Put ½ cup powdered whole milk into a bath bag with ½ cup dried chamomile flowers. Toss into a warm bath or hang from the faucet as the tub fills.
Fresh Method: Take 1 cup cold whole milk or cream out of the refrigerator and add a handful of fresh chamomile flowers (just-picked rose petals, calendula flowers, or other fresh blossoms are also good). Allow the herb to infuse at room temperature for several hours, then strain the milk into the tub as it fills.

Oatmeal Rose Bath: Put a handful of quick-cooking oats and a handful of dried rose petals into a bath bag to make a sweet-smelling, skin-soothing bath. For a milkier bath, you can also try powdering the rolled oats first in a coffee or spice grinder.

Resistance Boosting Bath: Fill the bath bag with a combination of fresh herbs including fresh thyme, fresh lavender flowers and leaves, fresh mint, and the grated rind of a lemon. Put the bag in the bath as it fills. Then squeeze the juice out of the lemon into the tub and swish to mix before you get in. To increase potency, add a few drops of essential oils of lavender and/or eucalyptus.

Quick Herbal Bath: Begin with hot water only. Add a half dozen herbal tea bags. Turn off the water and allow the tea bags to steep for five or ten minutes, then fill the tub the rest of the way with water that is a comfortable temperature for you.
    Cool baths (not cold! cold baths can cause dangerous shocks

to the system) are stimulating and help reduce body temperature during extremely hot and humid weather. One drop of peppermint essential oil or a bath bag filled with fresh mint placed in a cool or tepid bath can rejuvenate wilted kids or adults on a muggy summer day.

Bubble Baths

Kids love bubble baths, but most mass-market products are made with cheap, irritating ingredients, artificial dyes, and synthetic perfumes that, for little girls especially, can cause urinary tract infections or for both sexes can cause skin rashes. Watch out for sodium lauryl sulfate, which is a harsh surfactant (sodium laureth sulfate is milder, especially when combined with buffering agents), and sodium chloride, which is salt, used as a cheap thickener, in the ingredient lists, as well as the above-mentioned dyes and fragrances.

For occasional use, you can make your own bubble bath using a mild, unscented baby shampoo and a few drops of essential oil if you want an aromatherapeutic dimension.

Pink Princess Bubble Bath: My eldest daughter went through a few years of insisting that everything she had or did somehow be associated with the color pink. I know that it was probably not politically correct to indulge her, but she's eight years old now, and it's over. Well, mostly over. If you want to impress a pink-loving little girl and get her into the bathtub without endangering her genitourinary health, try mixing 1 tablespoon of fresh beet juice (one smallish beet through the juicer) with 2 tablespoons of mild, unscented bubble bath. You'll create a thick frosting of white or slightly pink bubbles with pink water underneath. It's a Pink Princess dream come true.

Unfortunately, natural sources that can color bathwater are fairly limited. I know that turmeric could be used as a natural coloring to create a *Golden Prince Bubble Bath* variation, but having a boy child of my own, and knowing the American male propensity for scatological humor, yellow bathwater might well remind them of something else.

Flower Essences in the Bath

The bathtub is also a great place to use flower essences, either those you have purchased or those you've created yourself. They can be added to an herb or essential oil blend or dropped into the water all by themselves to add a balancing emotional or spiritual dimension to your healing bath.

CHAPTER EIGHT

BEDTIME

There was never a child so lovely but his mother was glad to get him asleep.

—Ralph Waldo Emerson (1803–1882)

S tories are medicine. Both the act of telling a story and actively listening to a story as it is told have tremendous healing potential. Among ancient and aboriginal peoples, stories not only filled the long, dark nights of winter; they communicated important information about tribal history and culture, social expectations, and spiritual beliefs. Stories have always served to provide a framework of meaning, giving order to the chaos of the surrounding world and the variety of experiences human beings are likely to encounter there. Certain archetypes and story themes are found in so many and such geographically diverse cultures, that they hint at a common primordial origin. Keeping ancient stories alive is one way of keeping ourselves connected with our own remote and sacred beginnings. For this reason, a number of traditional stories from aboriginal cultures are included here.

Bedtime rituals are not only bonding times; they set the scene for that most precious and irreplaceable healing elixir, a good night's sleep. As mentioned in the previous chapter, for busy, working parents, bathtime and bedtime can be the best times of our day, as we slow down and unwind to simply be with our children. Mornings are so often hectic, getting everyone out the door for work or school. A child's afternoons are usually filled with homework and friends and extracurricular activities. Not until the end of the day do we have our children to ourselves again. With a soothing bedtime back massage, a story, a poem, or a fragrant foot rub later, we find ourselves pleasantly reconnected with what matters most in a family: each other. This sense of connectedness is integral to the experience of optimal health.

The Maui stories, told since time immemorial throughout the Pacific Islands, are believed to be among the oldest stories on Earth. Variations of these stories are told in Polynesia, New Zealand, Samoa, Fiji, and the Hawaiian Islands and are believed to originate from the first Pacific Islanders, who originally migrated from ancient Babylon and India. Maui is a hero whose mother was mortal but whose father was a supernatural being. His mother rejected him at first, already having four hungry sons to take care of. Not wanting the responsibility of a fifth son, she tied the baby up with a strand of her long hair and threw him into the ocean. But the sea god recognized Maui as part divine and sent the jellyfish to buoy him up, and warm waves to rock him and carry him back to shore. There Maui grew up, sustained by the sea, who brought him everything he needed. Maui, like Hercules, is remembered for the seven miraculous feats he performed. Here is the story of one of them.

Maui Raises Up the Sky

ave you ever wondered why leaves are flat? Think about it. The leaves of trees, blades of grass, even petals of flowers—all flat. They got this way because, in the beginning, the sky was pressed tightly up against the earth, and as the trees, plants, and flowers grew, they were squeezed flat in that narrow little space. There was not even enough room to stand up in, and people had to crawl around on their hands and knees to get from one place to another. Most people just accepted this, because, after all, it was just the way things were. But Maui was different. He got to wondering if there might not be some way to change things.

So he went to visit his grandmother, who lived on the mountain of Kahaleakala, which in Hawaiian means "House of the Sun," because that's where the sun comes from when it rises up each morning. Maui's grandmother listened to him and blessed him for having such an idea. She was an old woman, and her back hurt her from having to stoop as she walked around in that

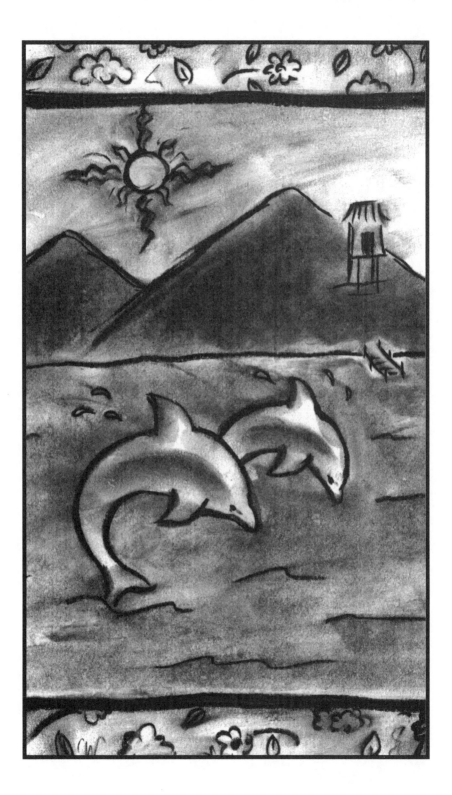

narrow little space between heaven and earth. She drew a magic tattoo on Maui's arm, which gave him superhuman strength. She made a magic potion for him and gave it to him to drink from a hollowed-out gourd.

When Maui was finished drinking, he felt incredible strength rising within himself. Wedging his shoulders against the low-hanging blue ceiling of the sky, he pushed with his back, with all his might. At first nothing happened. Maui braced his feet against the Earth and pushed again. Suddenly the sky gave way, arching above him. Trees sprang up straight from where the sky had been pinning them down, as did flowers, bushes, and plants. Maui's grandmother sighed with delight as she straightened her tired and aching body. She reached up with her hands as high as she could and wiggled her fingers in the open space above her head, something no one had ever done before.

Then Maui reached down from the mountaintop and picked up the edges of the sky that were still sticking to the ocean. He lifted them up high, on a level with the sky above the mountain. The curious dolphins poked their noses out of the water, for the first time without bumping into anything. What happened? they wondered among themselves. Where was the sky? "Maui," the waves whispered. "Maui has raised the sky." The dolphins leapt up above the surface of the water, trying to see Maui where he stood upon Kahaleakala, tucking up the last bits of blue. Higher and higher the dolphins leapt, chattering joyfully among themselves.

And to this day the sky remains up high where Maui put it, and the dolphins still jump out of the water, hoping to catch a glimpse of him. Sometimes the clouds sneak down from the sky and move in close to the Earth, bringing storms and rain. But they never stay for very long, because they know that if Maui caught them, his mighty arms would throw them so hard and so far that they would never find their way back again.

Here is another very old Hawaiian tale. Rainbows and their ephemeral beauty figure prominently in many ancient stories, from the biblical account of Noah's Ark to the Rainbow Bridge legends of American Indians. Children spend many happy hours drawing rainbows, which works of art then go on to festoon many a refrigerator gallery. The bright, momentary arc of color that suddenly appears after a rain seems to whisper a healing message of joy and hope as we pause for a moment to watch in wonder wherever and whenever a rainbow appears.

The Rainbow Princess

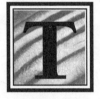

The lush, tropical islands of Hawaii were formed by volcanic eruptions of lava, smoothed by the washing waves of the sea. On one of the islands, deep chasms slash the surface of the land. In the old days, the only way the people could travel across the island was by means of knotted rope ladders made from jungle vines or twisted fibers. One day, a young couple was journeying across the island. The mother held her young baby against her with one arm as she used her other hand to climb up the rope ladder. They had almost reached the top of the chasm when, to the mother's horror, the baby slipped from her grasp and fell down, down, past the trees and vines that clung to the steep sides of the narrow opening. Within moments the baby was gone from sight, presumably dashed to pieces on the sharp cliffs or the rocks below. Believing the baby was dead, the mother and father climbed the rest of the way to the top, where they wept and consoled each other for the loss of their only child.

Unbeknownst to them, there was a waterfall halfway down the chasm, and the spirit of the water had heard the infant's frightened cries as she fell. The spirit of the waterfall called to the sun, and suddenly a rainbow appeared. Instead of landing on the jagged rocks at the bottom of the canyon, the baby slid safely

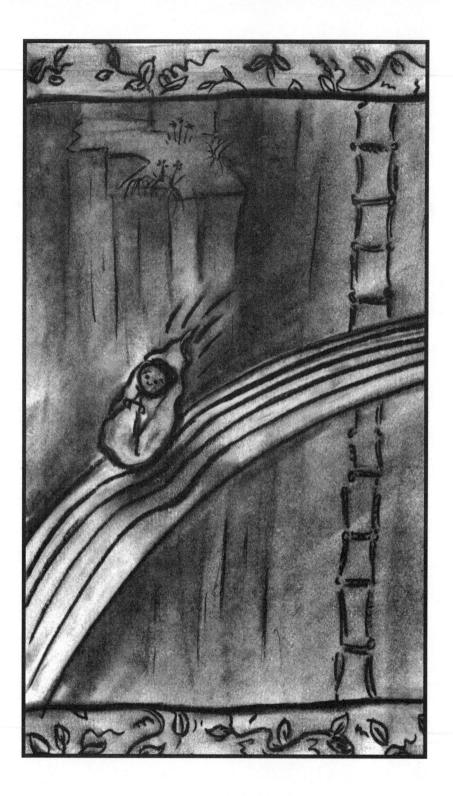

down the rainbow, through the waterfall, then rolled onto a ledge at the waterfall's side. Cared for by the spirits and creatures of the canyon, the baby grew up to be a beautiful young woman.

One day, as the girl washed herself in the clear, cold spray of the waterfall, she was spotted by a handsome young hunter. He stood and watched her for a long time, thinking she was the loveliest girl he had ever seen. Rainbows twirled around her neck and wrists, gleaming like jewelry. She sang as she combed out her long, glossy hair. Finally the young man could keep silent no more. "Who are you?" he cried, his heart leaping wildly in his chest. But when she saw him she only laughed and laughed. "Come back when you know my name!" she called. The young man decided he would climb up to her and introduce himself. But the cliff was steep and straight, and there was nothing to hang on to, not even the smallest outcropping where he could gain a foot- or handhold. Again and again he went back to the same spot, as near as he could approach her. But every time he called for her she laughed and paid no attention to him. Meanwhile, his heart had grown so full of love for her that he could not rest, and he could not think about anything else. There was nothing left for him to do but to find out her name.

The young man journeyed from island to island, asking about the rainbow princess in every village, at every hut, but no one knew who he was talking about, and none could tell him her name. He asked the fishermen as they unloaded their nets. He asked the chiefs and the women and the children. Without knowing it, he even asked the girl's parents, now grown old and childless. "My daughter would have been of such an age, and just as beautiful," the old woman said sadly, "but, as a baby, she was taken from my arms." Finally there was no one left to ask, and so, exhausted and dejected, the young man went home.

For lack of food and sleep, the young man had grown lean and gaunt. His grandmother, noticing his suffering, asked him what was wrong. Head bowed, the young man told her of the rainbow princess, of her great beauty and his love for her, of how she lived high on a cliff beside a waterfall out of his reach, and how she laughed at him when he tried to speak to her. "She has told me to come back when I know her name," the young man said with a heavy sigh. "But I have traveled to every island, and asked every man, woman, and child, and no one knows her. No one can tell me her name."

His grandmother was silent for a long moment. Then, smiling gently, she said, "Do as I say." The young man listened, and thanked her. As soon as the sun came up, he made his way back to the waterfall. Standing on a rock outcropping on the opposite side of the chasm, he called for the rainbow princess. Laughing, she stepped out through the mist and stood at the edge of the cliff, rainbow wisps twining over her shoulders and through her hair. "Oo ah," the young man sang to her, just as his grandmother had instructed him. "Oo ah. Oo ah." (This is the Hawaiian word for "rain.") Looking surprised, the young woman stopped laughing. Her eyes met his, and a rainbow bridge suddenly sprang across the chasm. Stepping onto the rainbow, the beautiful rainbow princess slid safely across and into his waiting arms.

In ancient Mayan and American Indian traditions, the hunter shows his respect and appreciation for a deer's sacrifice by making an offering and an apology for killing it to fill his need. In this ancient tale of India, the situation is reversed, and an important lesson is revealed about what it means to be a leader.

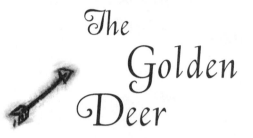

The Golden Deer

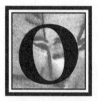nce, in ancient India, there lived a rajah who loved venison meat. He was constantly going out to hunt for deer, and every time he went, he called the men of the village to go with him. After a while the village women started to get upset, because the men were always out hunting with the rajah, and they never had time to finish their work. So the women got together and fenced in a large forest, with plenty of grass growing in it and a stream running through. Then they went out and captured as many deer as they could find and brought them back to live in their forest. The women fed the deer and fattened them up so that their meat was rich and tender. Once they had everything the way they wanted it, they created a padlock with a golden key. Bringing the plumpest, healthiest deer from their forest, they presented the golden key to the rajah and invited him to hunt there at his pleasure. The rajah gave the deer to his cook, who made a delicious venison roast from it. Delighted, the rajah went the very next day to hunt in the deer forest.

There were two tribes of deer in the forest. The golden deer were fine and large, with coats the color of spun gold and antlers that gleamed in the sunlight. The brown deer were smaller but had fine tails and horns like ivory. The first deer the rajah saw

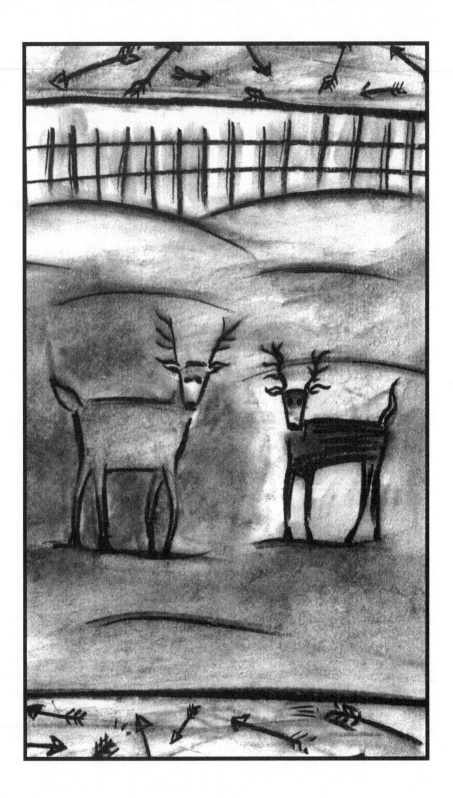

was the king of the golden deer. Recognizing another ruler when he saw him, the rajah granted the golden deer king his life. The second deer the rajah saw that day was the king of the brown deer. Also recognizing his royalty, the rajah granted the brown deer king his life as well. The third deer the rajah came upon he killed with his bow and arrow, and took it back to his palace for his cook to prepare for dinner.

The rajah hunted in the deer forest nearly every day. The deer knew what he came there for, and when they saw him, they were very much afraid. Sometimes they would run when they saw him, and the rajah would have to shoot arrows at five or six deer before hitting one with a mortal blow. Often the deer who were only wounded got sick and died of their injuries. The two deer kings, worried about how many of their people were being hurt and killed, got together and made the following plan: each of the deer tribes would take a turn offering one of their members to the king. This way, many lives could be saved and fewer deer would be hurt. All the deer in each tribe were given a number, and when their number was called, it was their day to die. The chosen deer would offer itself by standing directly in the rajah's path when he appeared, making the hunt easy and preventing unnecessary injuries. One day it would be a golden deer, the next day a brown deer. And so it went, and everyone was satisfied.

Until one day it was the turn of a brown doe who had just had her fawn. She went to the brown deer king and begged to be spared. "Please, my king," she asked. "If I die today my fawn will die also, because he is not yet old enough to live on his own. Please wait until my fawn can live on his own, and then I will gladly take my turn to die for my people." The brown deer king refused. "It is the law," he told her. "It is the agreement we made with the golden deer people. I cannot go back on my word."

Distraught, the brown deer mother went to the golden deer king and told him her story. His great eyes flashed like emeralds as he listened. "No law can have meaning without compassion," he told her. "Return to your child."

The next day, when the rajah entered the forest to hunt, he was surprised to see the king of the golden deer appear before him. "What are you doing here?" the rajah asked. "I have already spared your life." "I give my life freely," the golden deer king replied. The rajah looked over the golden deer king, at his sleek, glistening coat, and fine strong flesh. What a meal he would

173

make, enough for a feast! The rajah pulled back his arrow, taut against the bowstring. But before he released the arrow, he asked again, "Why? Why are you here?" The golden deer king told him that it was a brown deer mother's turn to die, and as it would not be fair of him to ask any of his own subjects to take the place of the deer from the other tribe, he could only offer himself.

The rajah put down his bow and arrow and was ashamed. He had not realized until that moment that the deer of the forest were capable of such thoughts and feelings. "Go back to your people," the rajah told the golden deer king, "and tell them I will hunt them no more." The golden deer king went free, and the rajah never ate venison meat again.

This is a story from the Cherokee tribe of American Indians. I found this story on the Internet in a large collection of traditional American Indian stories. I am very thankful to Darren Christmas, who put up the site, for his permission to use some of these wonderful old stories. He invites you to visit his Web page, where you can read all of them:
http://www.geocities.com/RainForest/5292/index.html.
His e-mail address is <Dinetah@flex.net>
I encourage you to visit. Many beautiful discoveries await you there.

Where Medicine Came From

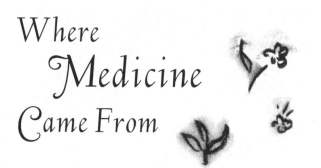

 t one time, animals and people lived together in peace and talked with each other. But when mankind began to multiply rapidly, the animals were crowded into forests and deserts. Man began thoughtlessly to destroy the animals for their skins and their fur, not only for the food people needed. Animals resented being treated this way by those who had once been their friends, and they decided they would have to punish mankind.

The bear tribe met in council with Old White Bear, their chief. Some of the bears got up and spoke about mankind's horrible wars, and a war was decided upon as just punishment. Chief Old White Bear suggested that man's own weapon, the bow and arrow, be used against him. All the bears agreed. They set about making bows and arrows, and one of the bears sacrificed himself to make bowstrings. When the first bow was finished, the bear's long claws got in the way, so that the arrow would not shoot properly. One bear offered to cut his claws, but Chief Old White Bear would not allow him to do it. Without his claws, the bear would not be able to climb trees to find food or reach safety. The bear might starve.

175

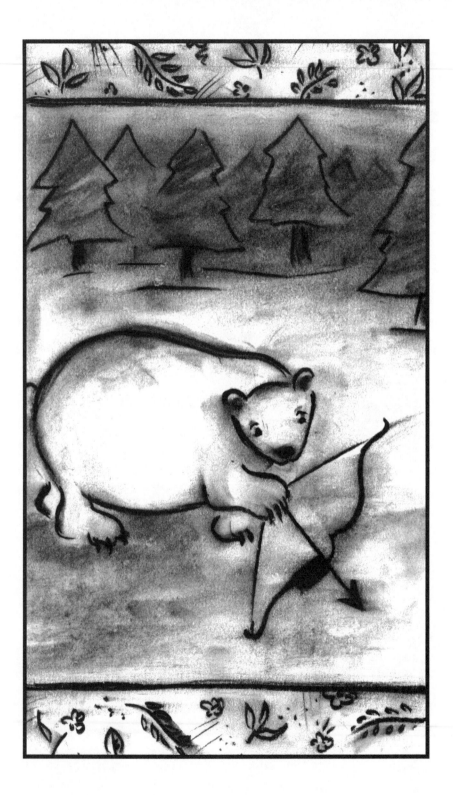

Then Chief Little Deer called together the deer tribe council. They decided that any Indian hunters who killed deer without asking for pardon should be afflicted with a painful disease, rheumatism, in their joints. Chief Little Deer sent a message to his nearest neighbors, the Cherokee Indians. "From now on, your hunters must first offer a prayer to the deer before killing him," said the messenger. "You must ask the deer's pardon, and tell him that you are sorry but the hunger of your tribe forces you to kill him. Otherwise, a terrible disease will come to the hunter."

So, from then on, when a deer is killed by an Indian hunter, Chief Little Deer will run to the spot and ask the slain deer's spirit, "Did you hear the hunter's prayer for pardon?" If the deer spirit answers yes, all is well, and Chief Little Deer goes back to his cave. But if the answer is no, Chief Little Deer follows the hunter home and strikes him with the terrible disease of rheumatism, which makes it impossible for him to hunt again.

Then the fishes and reptiles held a council together and decided that they would haunt any Cherokee Indians who tormented them, by making them have hideous dreams and nightmares. If a Cherokee Indian bothered fish, snakes, or lizards, he would have terrible dreams until he promised to stop.

But the plants stayed friendly to mankind. They had a council of their own, and each tree, shrub, herb, grass, and moss agreed to be a cure for each of the diseases that the animals and insects were coming up with as revenge against mankind. Ever after, if the Cherokee Indians went to their healer and he wasn't sure what to do, he would talk with the spirits of the plants. They always told him a remedy for mankind's diseases.

This was the beginning of plant medicine among the Cherokee Indian nation, a long, long, time ago.

Why the Opossum's Tail Is Bare

I t must be remembered that the animals that appear in Indian myths and legends are not the same as those that exist now. When the world began, animals were much bigger, stronger, and more clever than their present counterparts, but, because people treated them so badly, these animals left the earth and took the rainbow path to Galunlati, the Sky Land, where they live today. The animals that came after them—those we know today—are only poor, weak imitations of those first creatures.

In the beginning, before all this happened, all living things—men, animals, plants, and trees—spoke the same language and behaved in much the same way. Animals, like people, were organized into tribes. They had chiefs, lived in houses, held councils and ceremonies.

Back then, many animals were so different that we would not recognize them today. The rabbit, for example, was fierce, bold, and cunning and loved to play tricks on the other animals. It was because of the rabbit's tricks that the deer lost his sharp, wolflike teeth, the buzzard his handsome topknot of feathers, and the opossum his long, bushy tail.

Opossum was very proud of his tail, which, in those days, was covered with thick, black fur. He spent long hours cleaning and brushing it. He loved it so much that he wrote songs and poems about how beautiful it was. Sometimes when he walked through the village, he carried his tail erect, like a banner rippling in the breeze. At other times he swept it down low behind him, like a train. It was useful as well as beautiful, for when Opossum laid down to sleep, he tucked it under him to make a soft bed, and in cold weather he folded it over his body to keep himself warm.

Rabbit was very jealous of Opossum's magnificent tail. He, too, had once had a long bushy tail, but, during the course of a

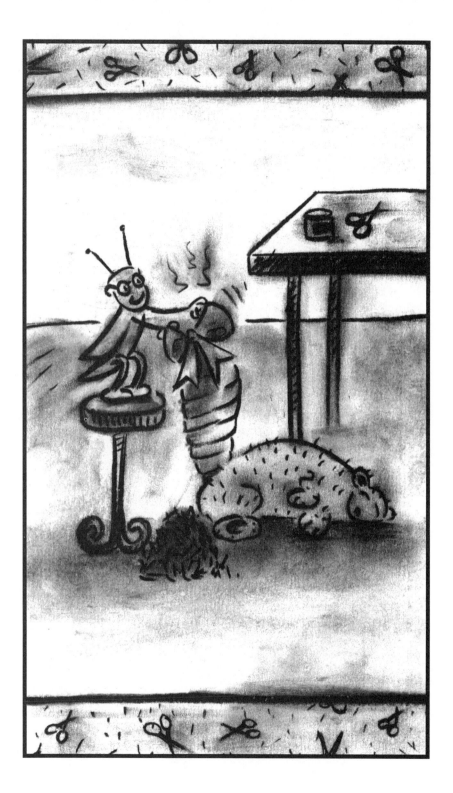

fight with Bear, he had lost most of it, and now he had only a short, fluffy tail. The sight of Opossum strutting around in front of the other animals, swirling his tail ostentatiously, filled Rabbit with rage. He made up his mind to play a trick on Opossum at the first opportunity.

At this time, when the animals still lived harmoniously together, each animal had a special job and duty to perform. Thus Frog was leader in the council and Rabbit, because of his speed, was appointed to carry messages and announcements to the others.

As was their custom from time to time, the animals decided to hold a great council to discuss important matters. Rabbit, as usual, was given the task of delivering the invitations. Councils were also occasions for feasting and dancing, and Rabbit saw a way of bringing about Opossum's downfall.

When Rabbit arrived with news of the meeting, Opossum was sitting by the door of his lodge, engaged in his favorite activity—grooming his tail. "I come to call you to the great council tomorrow, brother Opossum," said Rabbit. "Will you attend and join in the dance?"

"Only if I am given a special seat," replied the conceited Opossum, carefully smoothing some untidy hairs at the tip of his tail. "After all," he went on, grinning pointedly at Rabbit, "I have such a beautiful long tail that I ought to be sitting where everyone can see and admire it."

Rabbit was so angry he could hardly speak, but, ignoring the jibe, he said, "But of course, brother Opossum! I will personally see to it that you have the best seat in the council lodge, and I will also send someone to dress your tail specially for the dance!"

Opossum was delighted by this suggestion, and Rabbit left him singing the praises of his tail even more loudly than usual. Next, Rabbit went to the cricket, whom Indians call "the barber," because of his fame as an expert hair-cutter. Cricket listened with growing amazement as Rabbit recounted his conversation with Opossum. Like all the other animals, he found Opossum's vanity and arrogance very tiresome. He began to protest, but Rabbit held up a paw and said, "Wait a moment. I have a plan, and I need your help. Listen . . ." And he dropped his voice as he told Cricket what he wanted him to do.

Early next morning, Cricket arrived at Opossum's door and presented himself, saying he had been sent by Rabbit to prepare the famous tail for the council that evening. Opossum made himself comfortable on the floor and stretched out his tail. Cricket began to comb it gently. "I will wrap this red ribbon around your tail as I comb it," he explained, "so that it will stay smooth and neat for the dance tonight."

Opossum found Cricket's ministrations so soothing that he fell asleep. He didn't wake up until Cricket was tying the final knot in the red ribbon, which now completely covered his tail. *I will keep it bound up until the very last moment,* thought Opossum gleefully. *How envious the others will be when I finally reveal it in all its beauty!*

That evening, his tail still tightly wrapped in the red ribbon, Opossum marched into the council lodge and was led to his special seat by a strangely obsequious Rabbit.

Soon it was time for the dancing to take place. The drums and rattles began to sound. Opossum stood up, untied the ribbon from his tail, and stepped proudly into the center of the dance floor. He began to sing one of the songs he had made up about it.

"Look at my beautiful tail!" he sang. "See how it sweeps the ground!"

There was a loud shout from the audience, and some of the animals began to applaud. "How they admire me!" thought Opossum, and he continued to dance and sing loudly. "See how my tail gleams in the firelight!"

Again everyone shouted and cheered. Opossum hesitated a moment. Was there possibly a hint of mockery in their voices? No, it couldn't be. He continued dancing.

"My tail is stronger than the eagle's, more lustrous than the raven's!"

At this the animals shrieked so loudly that Opossum stopped in his tracks and looked at them. To his astonishment and chagrin, they were all laughing, some leaning weakly on each other's shoulders, others rolling on the ground in their mirth. Several of them were pointing at his tail.

Bewildered, Opossum looked down. To his horror, he saw that his tail, his beautiful, thick, glossy tail, was now bald and scaly-looking, like the tail of a lizard. Nothing remained of its former glory. While pretending to comb it, the wily Cricket had snipped off every single hair.

Opossum was so ashamed and embarrassed that he couldn't utter a sound. Instead, he rolled over helplessly on his back, grimacing with embarrassment, just as opossums still do today, when taken by surprise.

How the Chipmunk Got His Stripes

ong ago when animals could talk, a bear was walking along. Now it has always been said that bears think very highly of themselves. Since they are big and strong, they are certain that they are the most important of the animals.

As this bear went along, turning over big logs with his paws to look for food to eat, he felt very confident, very sure of himself. "There is nothing I cannot do," said this bear.

"Is that so?" said a small voice. Bear looked down. There was a little chipmunk looking up at Bear from its hole in the ground.

"Yes," Bear said, "that is true indeed." He reached out one huge paw and rolled over a big log. "Look how easily I can do this. I am the strongest of all the animals. I can do anything. All the other animals are afraid of me."

"Can you stop the sun from rising in the morning?" asked the Chipmunk.

Bear thought for a moment. "I have never tried that," he said. "But I'm sure I could do it. Yes, I am sure I could stop the sun from rising."

"You are sure?" said Chipmunk.

"I am sure," said Bear. "Tomorrow morning the sun will not rise. I, Bear, have said so." Bear sat down facing the east to wait. Behind him the sun set for the night, and still he sat there. Chipmunk went into his hole and curled up in his snug little nest, chuckling about how foolish Bear was. All through the night Bear sat. Finally the first birds started their songs and the east glowed with the light that comes before the sun.

"The sun will not rise today," said Bear. He stared hard at the glowing light. "The sun will not rise today."

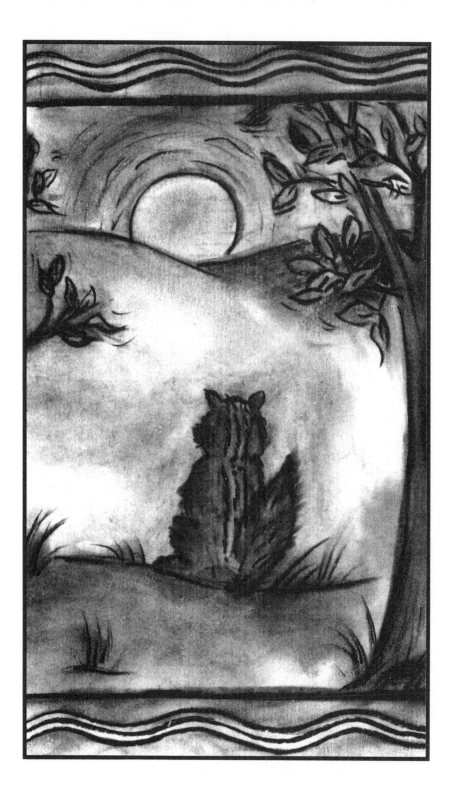

However, the sun rose, just as it always had. Bear was very upset, but Chipmunk was delighted. He laughed and laughed. "Sun is stronger than Bear," said Chipmunk, twittering with laughter. Chipmunk was so amused that he came out of his hole and began running around Bear in circles, singing this song:

"The sun came up,
The sun came up.
Bear is angry,
But the sun came up."

While Bear sat there looking very unhappy, Chipmunk ran around and around, singing and laughing until he was so weak that he rolled over on his back. Then, quicker than the leap of a fish from a stream, Bear shot out one big paw and pinned Chipmunk to the ground. "Perhaps I cannot stop the sun from rising," growled Bear, "but you will never see another sunrise."

"Oh, Bear," said Chipmunk. "Oh, oh, oh, you are the strongest, you are the quickest, you are the best of all of the animals. I was only joking." But Bear did not move his paw.

"Oh, Bear," Chipmunk said, "you are right to kill me. I deserve to die. Just please let me say one last prayer to the Creator before you eat me up."

"Say your prayer quickly," said Bear. "Your time to walk the Sky Road has come!"

"Oh, Bear," said Chipmunk, "I would like to die. But you are pressing down on me so hard that I cannot breathe. I can hardly squeak. I do not have enough breath to say a prayer. If you would just lift your paw a little, just a little bit, then I could breathe. And I could say my last prayer to the Maker of all, to the one who made great, wise, powerful Bear, and the foolish, weak, little Chipmunk."

Bear lifted up his paw. He lifted it up just a little bit. That little bit, though, was just enough. Chipmunk squirmed free and ran for his hole as quick as the blink of an eye. Bear swung his big paw at the little chipmunk as it darted away. He was not quick enough to catch him, but the very tips of his long claws scraped along Chipmunk's back, leaving three pale scars.

To this day, all chipmunks wear those scars as a reminder to them of what happens when one animal makes fun of another.

The next two are stories I made up at bedtime for my own children. I include them to encourage you to do the same.

The Rainbow Angels

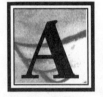 long, long time ago, before there were any people, there was a rainbow that stretched between heaven and earth. Now this rainbow wasn't like the rainbows that you see today, so faint and faraway. This was a strong, sturdy rainbow, as solid as a bridge or a playground slide. And in fact, that's what the angels used it for.

Because it's very quiet in heaven. Angels have wings, so there are no cars or buses, no planes or trains The music is soft, and angels speak in whispers. Most of the time that's fine. But every once in a while, even angels get the feeling that they want to shout out loud, or run around, or jump into a mud puddle. When they wanted to do something like that, they would sneak off and slide down the rainbow to the Earth, which was like a wonderful playground for them.

There were no people or animals on earth then, only trees, big forests, and fields of flowers. It rained a lot, so there were lots of mud puddles to play in. As the angels slid down the rainbow, some of the color would rub off on them. Depending on which color stripe they slid down, they would be that color when they hit the ground. Imagine what a bright and colorful sight it was: red angels, purple angels, blue angels, green angels, orange angels, yellow angels, indigo angels, all chasing each other around the trees and through the flowers, yelling and yelling and singing and dancing, and jumping into the mud puddles, getting dirty and having a wonderful time.

When it came time to return to heaven, the angels would rinse off the mud and the color in the nearest pond or stream. The sun would dry them, then they'd walk back up the rainbow very carefully, holding up their wings so they wouldn't drag in the

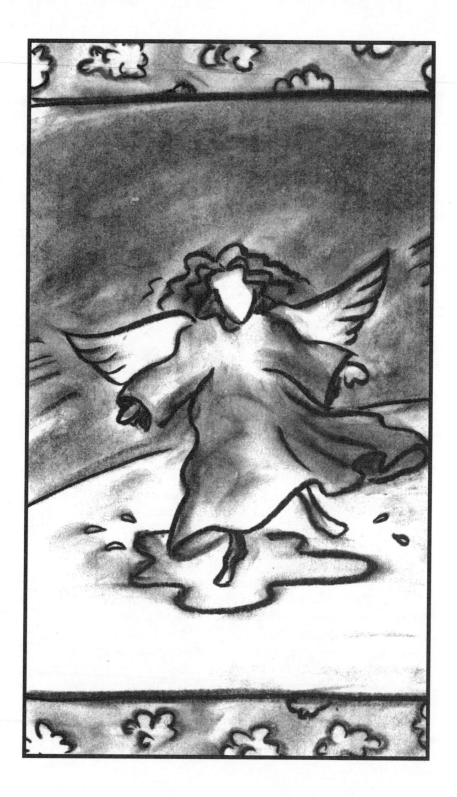

color. But they weren't really fooling anyone, because if you looked carefully, you could see their little colored footprints all over the clouds.

But one day winter came to the Earth and stayed for thousands of years. This was the Ice Age. The Earth turned white, covered over with ice and snow, and the rainbow froze solid as an ice cube. Still the angels came down to play on the frozen planet. They skated down or slid along the frozen stripes. Not as much color rubbed off on them now, so they were only lightly tinted, yellowish, reddish, purplish, when they hit the ground. They skated and threw snowballs and whooshed down the snowbanks. They laid down and moved their arms and legs, leaving pale pastel imprints when they got up—the first snow angels.

Gradually it got warmer, and the snow began to melt. Now there were more mud puddles to play in than ever! Some of the angels had such a good time splashing around in them, and watching the new spring buds and flowers, that they stayed down on the Earth for longer and longer periods of time. As the frozen rainbow began to thaw, it was getting slick and slippery, and getting back up to heaven was becoming more difficult. And then one day, a terrible cracking noise was heard from the rainbow. And then another CRACK! And another!

Frightened, some of the angels ran into the forest and hid. Others ventured out to see what was happening. As they looked up, a big chunk of rainbow fell onto the Earth, causing the ground to rumble and shake. Like ice breaking up on a river in springtime, the frozen rainbow was shattering and falling in pieces all over the Earth. Some of the chunks fell into the mud puddles and splashed the angels who were watching until they turned brown. Others kept the reddish, yellowish, or pinkish tints they had from sliding down the rainbow. Some played in the sun so long that they turned almost black.

Knowing that they couldn't get back to heaven anymore, the stranded angels decided to make the best of things. They put away their wings and became the first human beings. Even today, if you look very closely at people, you will see a little bit of rainbow color tinting their skin. Even today, from time to time, the ghost of that old rainbow slide still appears, especially in the spring, after the rain. And when we see a rainbow, it makes us happy, because it reminds us of the time when the Earth was our playground and heaven was our home.

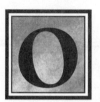

The Child Who Was Afraid
of the Night

nce there was a child who was afraid of the night. This child's mother had tried everything to get her to sleep. She tried nice warm baths and bedtime stories, night lights and backrubs. Every night the mother did these things, and she sat next to her child on the edge of the bed until the child grew sleepy and dozed off. The mother would kiss her child on the forehead, tiptoe out, and go to her own bed to sleep, because like most mothers, she was very tired at the end of the day.

But every night, shortly after her mother left the room, the child would awaken, alone and afraid. The small glowing circle around the night-light seemed so tiny, and the night seemed so big, that soon the child would be yelling and crying. The mother would get up and go in to comfort the child. And no one was getting a decent night's sleep.

One day the Sun looked down. He saw the dark circles under their eyes and the way they yawned over breakfast and fell asleep in the middle of whatever they were doing in the afternoon. That evening as he was setting, the Sun paused to have a word with the Moon, who was just coming up. "What's the matter with those two?" the Sun asked. "All day long I shine and shine, and do you think they appreciate it? No! They can barely stay awake."

"It's the child," said the Moon, her round face beginning to glow in the darkening sky. "The child is afraid of the night."

The Sun had his mouth open to reply, but just at that moment, he slipped under the horizon, and nothing more was said. But the Night had been listening. As the Sun popped down to shine over one half of the planet, the Night pulled his big, dark blanket embroidered with stars over the other half. *Why?* he wondered. *Why would a child be afraid of me?* He resolved to find out.

Once it was dark, he went to the house where the child lived and sat outside her window. He watched as the child's mother tucked her in. When the child became sleepy, the mother kissed

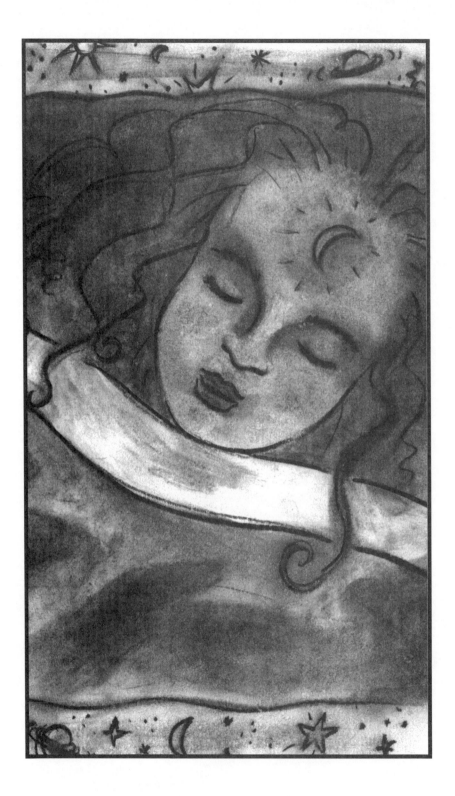

the child on the forehead, turned off the lamp, and turned on a night light. Then she tiptoed out of the room.

Leaning against the sill of the open window, watching the child sleep, the Night wondered again what it was about him that made the child so afraid. The Moon, looking over his shoulder, whispered into his ear, "It's because she doesn't understand. She doesn't know you. Human beings are afraid of what they don't understand."

Just at that moment, the child woke up. Seeing the Night leaning in through the window, she became very frightened. Her eyes grew big and round, and just as she was about to start screaming, a warm, gentle breeze blew into the room. A sweet fragrance came with it, like the perfume of a night-blooming jasmine. The child relaxed just a little, until she heard a dark, smoky voice, lower than a whisper. "Why do you fear me?"

The child wanted to scream again, but the breeze was so soft and warm, and its aroma so sweet, that she answered instead. "Well . . . because you're so big and I'm so small, and because when you're here, I can't see anything. I . . . I want you to go away."

The room grew still. Again the low voice whispered, "As you wish. But I want to be your friend. If you knew me, you wouldn't be afraid. Now, sleep." The Night moved away from the window, and the child laid down and went to sleep.

And so every night for the next week, as soon as the Sun popped below the horizon, the Night came and waited outside the child's window. Sometimes, when the child awakened, the Night would tell her stories of the stars and moon and planets, of how they came to be. Sometimes he told stories of animals and creatures who played in the dark as others did during the day. The child began to look forward to the Night's visits. The mother was happy to be getting a good night's sleep.

On his seventh visit, the Night came in through the window and sat on the end of the child's bed. "Come with me," he whispered in his dark, smoky voice. "I want to show you something." Taking the child's hand, the Night folded her in his warm, dark cloak, which was as soft as velvet. Together they floated, out through window and up into the dark sky.

Holding the Night's hand, the child flew laughing in a ring around the Moon. Together they danced among the stars. They watched from the treetops as deer came out of the forest and drank at the river's edge. The Night showed the child flowers that bloom only in the dark. Quick, darting bats flew by them, and, in the branches of a tree, they surprised a ghostly opossum. They raced with gossamer-winged moths, the nighttime butterflies. They joined in with coyotes howling at the Moon. They flew to the North Pole, and the Night spread his warm cloak over a glacier as they sat in quiet wonder watching the aurora borealis, the northern lights, a great kaleidoscope of color pulsing and swirling in the sky above the frozen tundra. "This is my night light," the Night said quietly.

"I never knew," the child whispered, snuggling deeper into his cloak. "I never knew you were so beautiful." Smiling, the Night looked down and saw that she had fallen asleep. Cradling her in his arms, he carried the child back to her bed, tucked her in, and, as he had seen her mother do, kissed her lightly on the forehead. And where he kissed her, there appeared, just for a moment, the faint silver imprint of a crescent moon.

From that time on, the child was no longer afraid of the Night. Both she and her mother slept quite well. The dark circles disappeared from under their eyes, and they stopped falling asleep in the middle of whatever they were doing in the afternoon, which made the Sun very happy. And sometimes, when the mother turned out the light and bent to kiss her child good night, she thought she could see a faint silvery something glowing on the child's forehead. But when she moved closer, there was nothing there.

CHAPTER NINE

MOTHER EARTH'S GUIDE *to* COMMON AILMENTS

he following are some suggestions for natural remedies to help alleviate common conditions. Always use common sense when it comes to your health and the health of your family. If symptoms persist for more than two days or worsen, contact a qualified medical practitioner. For dosages and cautions, please consult individual listings of the remedies suggested in previous chapters.

ACHES AND PAINS

For transitory discomfort, at the onset of illness or after overexertion, try some of the remedies listed below. If you experience frequent achiness or have a condition such as rheumatism or arthritis, a detoxifying regimen can help clean out your system. Aches and pains can also result when negative emotions are held in the body and not released; a talk with a friend or therapist can help immensely. Chronic or long-lasting pain can indicate a serious condition and should be diagnosed by a health care professional.

Herbs: Externally, macerated massage oils of **comfrey** or **St. John's Wort**; internally, **St. John's Wort, vervain, or white willow** in tea or tincture.

Homeopathics: Aconite, for aches that occur at the onset of flu; **Arnica,** for aches and pains resulting from bruising, a fall, overexertion, after surgery or dental work; **Apis,** for burning or constricting pains; **Bryonia,** for rheumatic or abdominal pains, or aches in the back, joints, or knees that get worse from movement; **Hypericum,** for pains resulting from nerve damage or blows to the spine; **Rhus tox,** for pains as a result of strain or heavy lifting, torn ligaments, sprains, aches that feel better after stretching or movement.

Flower Essences: Agrimony, for those who are in pain but put on a cheerful face; **Five Flower** or **Rescue Remedy,** for pains resulting from an accident or trauma, especially when accompanied by fear; **Sweet Chestnut,** for pain that seems unbearable to the point of anguish.

Essential Oils: Anti-inflammatory and analgesic essences include chamomile, lavender, or rosemary in bath, massage, or compresses; ginger, juniper, lavender, marjoram, or rosemary for aches and pains resulting from tension or fatigue; to improve circulation and alleviate stiffness, massage with a dilution of benzoin, black pepper, eucalyptus, or marjoram; for inflamed joints, chamomile (blue or Roman); for muscle pain, bay, birch, nutmeg, peppermint, or rosemary in bath, massage oil, or compress.

ATTENTION DEFICIT (HYPERACTIVITY) DISORDER (ADD/ADHD)

The incidence of ADD/ADHD has increased 500 percent over the last forty-five years. Nearly 10 percent of American children have been diagnosed with attention deficit, behavioral, or learning disorders. The National Institute of Mental Health has estimated that up to two million American children are affected, with boys being diagnosed with the disorder at a rate two to three times that of girls. Nearly 2 percent of school-age children, some six hundred thousand, are currently taking stimulant medication for ADD symptoms. The most common treatment is the prescription drug methylphenidate, best known by its trade name, Ritalin, which is manufactured by Ciba Pharmaceuticals. Dextramphetamine, marketed as Dexedrine, and pemoline, marketed as Cylert, are also used.

A famous study conducted in 1988 revealed that in Baltimore County, Maryland, there was a consistent doubling of the rate of medication treatment for hyperactive/inattentive students every four to seven years, starting in 1971 and peaking in 1987.[1] Following all the negative publicity that attended the results of this study, use of Ritalin there declined 39 percent by 1992. Yet the use of Ritalin and the controversy surrounding its use continue to grow.

ADHD is not a bona fide medical disease, or even a clearly defined behavioral problem. Its diagnosis is determined by vague and subjective guidelines, usually based on observations by teachers and parents. Some believe it is little more than a label conveniently applied to children who do not fit into a system that has not been designed with their optimal development in mind. However, the commonly recognized aggregate symptoms of inattention, moodiness, anxiety, disorganization, and impulsivity can have a profoundly negative impact on children and their families. According to Paul Wender, a professor of psychiatry at the University of Utah School of Medicine, who has researched ADD treatments for thirty years, "These kids are likely to abuse drugs, to fall afoul of the legal system. This is not a benign condition. This is the most common childhood psychiatric disease associated with serious consequences."

Although Ritalin or Dexedrine may have a calming effect, one 1990 summary of studies stated that such drugs "are not specific for hyperactive children; they have the same [calming] effect on everyone."[2] A follow-up study in Baltimore County concluded that 36 percent of all ADHD children who were taken off medication experienced "school maladjustment," which leaves 64 percent who apparently had no major adjustment problems.[3] No evidence exists to show that achievement levels in the classroom are improved by the use of these drugs. However, there is a body of evidence linking Ritalin and other stimulants to side effects such as headaches, insomnia, stunted growth, and nervous tics such as Tourette's syndrome.[4] Cylert has been associated with possible liver damage. The long-term effects of using these drugs on children have not been studied and are not known.

Stephen B. Edelson of the Environmental and Preventive Health Center of Atlanta is a medical doctor who has worked with many ADHD children. Citing several studies of ADHD undertaken over the last twenty years, he believes that the majority of cases are caused by an immune system defect, sensitivities to food additives, preservatives, chemicals, or inhalants, and heavy metal toxicity. Stressful or dysfunctional home situations can also contribute to the problem.

Specific nutritional deficiencies that can contribute to ADHD include calcium, magnesium, iodine, and iron deficiencies, and high serum copper. Low zinc and high copper metabolism is also linked to dyslexia. Following a comprehensive patient history, physical exam, and laboratory evaluation, Dr. Edelson has had good results treating ADHD cases with individualized nutritional supplements, dietary changes, and immunotherapy.

Essential fatty acid deficiencies, in particular omega-3, are also implicated in ADHD, especially in boys. Omega-3, which is primarily concentrated in the brain, is not made by the body and can be found in dietary sources such as soybean and flaxseed oils, cold-water fish such as salmon, mackerel, tuna, and herring, and walnuts. Its lack has been associated with dry skin and hair, dandruff, excessive thirst and urination, and ADHD symptoms such as anxiety, impulsivity, temper tantrums, insomnia, and learning disabilities in six- to twelve-year-old boys.

According to Dr. Edelson, "We place our children in classrooms for eight hours a day, five days a week. In those forty hours, they breathe in chemicals from carpets, paints, pesticides, toxic cleaning fluids, furniture, office machinery, etc. In addition, most schools are contaminated with molds. And if the building is more than twenty-five years old, you can add in the asbestos factor." Noting that in his experience, allergies are the most common cause of learning disabilities, he continues, "Alien chemicals, heavy metals, and contaminated air and water can cause an individual child's immune system to become damaged. This can cause sensitivities to certain foods, chemicals, preservatives, and molds. As a result, a child may develop a learning disability."

Dr. William Crook, author of *The Yeast Connection* and *Help for the Hyperactive Child*, adds the adverse effects of too much television and not enough exercise, overuse of antibiotics, and yeast overgrowth to the list of possible triggers for ADD/ADHD and associated learning disabilities. Although Ritalin can be very effective in controlling symptoms in as much as 80 percent of ADHD children, he notes that there are no long-term benefits to the child's normal development. Some studies indicate that there may also be more behavioral problems and substance abuse later in life for children who have taken Ritalin. Dr. Crook believes that 75 percent or more of ADHD children do not need Ritalin and can be effectively treated by natural means.

Allergic reactions can be mistaken for ADD/ADHD symptoms. Common allergens include tobacco smoke, synthetic perfumes, chemical cleaners and insecticides, as well as foods such as sugar, "fast" or processed foods in general, foods containing MSG, preservatives, artificial dyes, sweeteners, and/or flavors, milk, corn, chocolate or cocoa, eggs, wheat, soy, peanuts, and oranges. An "elimination diet" has been shown by a number of studies to be very effective in pinpointing food allergies that cannot be detected by allergy tests. Such a diet can be a lot of work but can yield truly valuable information. Start by keeping a written record of symptoms for at least three days before beginning the diet. Allergic symptoms may include inattentiveness, depression, tiredness, paleness, dark circles under the eyes, headaches, muscle aches, stomachaches, coughing or congestion, irritability, and overactivity. Then, for one to two weeks, eliminate the above-mentioned problem foods from the child's diet. Keep a record of symptoms during the diet and note any improvement. To find out which specific foods are the culprits, add the eliminated foods back into the diet one at a time and note any reactions. Allergic reactions may occur immediately, or up to twenty-four hours after. Nutrition can be augmented by the use of **blue-green algae** supplements. **Bee pollen** may also be useful if allergies are suspected.

ADD/ADHD kids need a lot of love and understanding, which their behavior can sometimes make difficult to give. A child who is having trouble at school and difficulty controlling moods and behavior often experiences feelings of self-hatred and low self-esteem, which can be exacerbated by punitive behavior on the part of an overtaxed parent. Extra hugs and positive attention can help. But don't forget to take care of yourself too, when you need it. See the suggestions under the heading "Stress."

The following suggestions are not a substitute for the guidance of a medical health professional. If you suspect your child has ADD/ADHD, consult with a physician.

Herbs: Calming herbs such as **chamomile, hops, passionflower, skullcap,** and **valerian** can be given in the form of tea or tincture; **gingko, gotu kola,** and **kelp** improve brain function; **alfalfa** helps cleanse the blood and is nutritious as well.

Homeopathics: Anacardium, for poor memory, low self-esteem, no patience, impulsiveness, refusal to do work, tendency to insult and swear, much better after eating; **Chamomilla,** when cranky, restless, colicky; **Graphites,** for smart-alecky behavior, laughter when reprimanded, teasing others, child may catch cold easily and tend to be overweight; **Nux vomica,** especially for boys who eat a poor diet, do not get enough fresh air or exercise, and exhibit sullen, angry, critical behavior; **Staphysagria,** for uncontrolled behavior, extreme sensitivity to what others think of them, loners, hypochondriacs, preoccupied with sex, may have history of sexual abuse.

Flower Essences: Aspen, for free-floating anxiety, cause not known; **Clematis,** for dreaminess, lack of focus; **Larch,** for lack of confidence, low self-esteem; **Mimulus,** for fear of known things, such as going to school or being ridiculed by others.

Essential Oils: Aromatic massage with calming essences can be useful to bring hyperactive kids "into their bodies." Try **chamomile, lavender, mandarin, neroli, rose.**

ALLERGIES

Allergic reactions include itchy, watery eyes, sneezing and runny nose, and in some cases skin reactions such as swelling and hives. Although it is not fully understood why some people develop allergies, allergies are generally recognized to be an overreaction by the immune system, which overmobilizes inappropriately to fight off a perceived invader. Certain precautions can be taken in the home, such as eliminating dust, artificial fragrances, and chemicals from the home environment. Make sure filters for air conditioners and furnaces are changed frequently. Pet hair and waste can also aggravate those who are susceptible. Eliminate sugary or processed foods from the diet. Avoid foods commonly known to aggravate allergies such as dairy products, chocolate, caffeine, nuts, eggs, wheat, shellfish, tomatoes, strawberries, citrus fruits, and additives such as artificial dyes and colors. Supplements such as vitamins A, B complex, C with bioflavonoids, essential fatty acids, acidophilus, calcium/magnesium, potassium, and tyrosine can also help relieve allergies.

Herbs: Angelica, to increase antibodies; **bee pollen,** in small amounts, to slowly build immunity to allergens; **burdock,** as a blood purifier; *Echinacea angustifolia,* short-term use, for allergies accompanied by bacterial infections; **eyebright,** internally or as an eyewash; **garlic,** a natural antibiotic and immune system enhancer; **ginger,** to aid in digestion, ½ ounce fresh ginger juice with a small amount of honey; **goldenseal,** a natural antibiotic; **elder flower, hyssop,** and **mullein,** for hayfever; **lemon,** fresh juice squeezed into warm water; **licorice,** anti-inflammatory, soothes mucous membranes; **lobelia,** to loosen congestion and relax spasms; **milk thistle,** to improve liver function; *Urtica dioica,* fresh leaf extract (suggested use: one month before allergy season, throughout allergy season, then stop one month after allergy season).

Homeopathics: Allium cepa, for sneezing symptoms accompanied by frontal headache, red, rubbed eyes, watery, burning discharge of mucus from the nose that improves in the open air and gets worse in a warm room; **Ambrosia,** for nasal discharge and itchy, watery eyes following exposure to ragweed; **Apis,** for itching, swelling, and puffiness that is worse at night and with heat; **Arsenicum,** for sneezing, rough breathing, burning discharge from nose and eyes that may be worse on the right side and after midnight; **Euphrasia,** for profuse burning tears that get worse in open air, watery nasal mucus that worsens at night, when lying down, and in the wind; **Natrum mur,** for spring and fall attacks of hay fever characterized by loss of sense of taste and smell, sneezing, watery nasal mucus and tears, worse in the morning, possibly accompanied by chapped lips and cold sores; **Nux vomica,** for sneezing, runny nose during the day becoming congestion at night, irritability, chills, worse indoors, better in the open air; **Pulsatilla,** for moody, sensitive children who crave affection and sympathy, runny nose turning into congestion at night, worse in warmth and while lying down, roof of the mouth may itch at night; **Sulfur,** for summer hay fever, worse from heat or sun, that may progress into asthma, reddened eyes and nose, burning, unpleasant-smelling nasal discharge, stuffed up indoors, runny nose outdoors.

Flower Essences: Crab Apple, the general cleansing remedy.

Essential Oils: To be used in the bath, as an inhalation, diffuser blend, or massage oil. **German chamomile,** for soothing of skin reactions or digestive disturbances; **Roman chamomile,** for stress relief, calming, and respiratory disturbances; **lavender,** a natural antibiotic and stress reliever; **melissa,** in dilutions of 1 percent or less, for allergies accompanied by skin problems or respiratory difficulties, especially where the chamomiles have not been effective; **rose,** for stress relief, skin reactions, and respiratory problems.

ANGER

Anger and its variations, such as rage, hatred, resentment, and hostility, are toxic emotions that have measurable, destructive effects on the human body. Anger held in the body can be experienced as abscesses and sores, aches and pains, fever, infections, inflammations, and depression. Chronic indulgence in negative emotions can result in damage to organs and tissues and a weakening and tearing down of the immune system. Often anger is the result of negative habits of thought and belief that have been learned, inherited, or acquired through unconscious repetition, in which case the habitual cultivation of opposite and positive emotions such as compassion, love, tenderness, and joy are the best long-term antidote. Meditation, prayer, active service, and conscious dwelling on positive thoughts can help retrain the mind, directing emotional response away from well-worn pathways. To break the pattern of the habitual anger response, the following can be very useful.

Herbs: Chamomile or **lavender flowers** are soothing and calming, fresh or dried, in bath or tea; **lemon balm,** fresh, as a tea or in the bath, is soothing and calming; **milk thistle,** to cleanse and strengthen the liver.

Homeopathics: Bryonia, for grumpy people who do not want company; **Chamomilla,** for anger or tantrums as a result of hypersensitivity, although the child may be comforted for a while by rocking or carrying; **Colocynthis,** for the easily offended, irritable, chronic complainer; **Nux vomica,** for the "poor loser" who may also be a rebel inclined to throwing tantrums; **Stramonium,** for wild, uncontrollable rage that may be accompanied by hallucinations, delusions, and foul language; **Staphysagria,** for those who are hypersensitive and easily offended and who hold deeply suppressed anger that tends to suddenly explode, particularly when there has been a history of sexual or physical abuse.

Flower Essences: Beech, for habitual anger that manifests as fault-finding and constant criticism; **Holly,** for anger held inside in the form of poisonous thoughts and feelings toward others such as jealousy, envy, suspicion, and revenge; **Impatiens,** for outbursts of anger due to impatience and irritation with others—a good remedy for those who "just can't wait" and who tend to grab at what they want, thus setting off arguments and violating the personal boundaries of others; **White Chestnut,** for uncontrollable, obsessive thinking in the aftermath of an argument, which may prevent letting go of anger.

Essential Oils: Ylang-ylang, a hypotensive essence, can be sniffed directly from the bottle to quiet the physiological turbulence anger creates in the body; **juniper,** to clear the air after an argument and to dispel negativity; **rose,** to open the heart and lovingly transform and elevate consciousness above the reach of negative emotion. Bouts of anger that erupt as a result of stress and nervous tension can respond well to stress-relieving essences such as **lavender, marjoram,** or **melissa,** or mood elevators such as **clary sage** or the **citruses.**

ANXIETY AND FEAR

Chronic anxiety and fear are particularly associated with the kidneys in subtle medicinal approaches and can be a predisposing factor in digestive problems, migraines, allergies, insomnia, and heart disease. Untreated, anxiety can tear down the body as quickly and surely as other toxic emotions such as anger or depression.

Herbs: Chamomile tea or bath; **kava kava** extract (not for lactating or pregnant women); **fresh lemon balm** tea or bath; **lobelia** extract or tincture; **passionflower,** a natural tranquilizer, is not appropriate for younger children.

Homeopathics: Aconite, for fear out of proportion to

circumstances, fear of dying of a minor ailment, easily startled, possibly with heart palpitations, tingling, or numbness in feet and hands, worse at night and in warm rooms, better in the fresh air, though not in a cold wind; **Argentum nitricum**, for fear of being alone, nervous diarrhea in fearful anticipation of some event, fearful delusions, impulsivity, hyperactivity, craving for sweets and salt; **Arsenicum album,** for fear to the point of anguish, extreme oversensitivity, frightening dreams or night terrors, worse after midnight; **Belladonna,** for night terrors, hallucinations, desire to bite or escape; **Borax,** for fear of downward motion, disinterest in learning, more cheerful after bowel movement; **Calcarea carbonica,** for anxiety and restlessness, worse at night, may see faces in nightmares, have bad reaction to milk while craving ice cream, eggs, salt, and inedible things like chalk, dirt, or pencil lead; **Gelsemium,** for stage fright, diarrhea, nervousness, and limpness; **Ignatia,** for emotional strain, grief, shock, fearfulness, hysteria, mood swings, very sensitive to tobacco smoke; **Lycopodium,** for apprehension and irritability worse from 4 P.M. to 8 P.M.; **Natrum phosphoricum,** for waking up at night and imagining footsteps or that a piece of furniture is a person, may be accompanied by canker sores and acid stomach, with creamy yellow coating on back of tongue or discharge from eyes, one ear red, hot, and itchy, often as a result of too much sugar; **Stramonium,** child may wake screaming from nightmares, be afraid of the dark, tunnels, water, drowning, or may have aversion to water touching the head, may be violent and suspicious, overreacting to small annoyances.

Flower Essences: Aspen, for feelings of dread, fear without a known cause; **Cherry Plum,** fear of losing control or going insane; **Mimulus,** for fears with known causes; **Red Chestnut,** for fear of what may happen to loved ones or others; **Rock Rose,** for extreme fear or terror, sometimes to the point of fainting or losing consciousness; **Five Flower** or **Rescue Remedy,** for fear resulting from an accident, shock, or trauma.

Essential Oils: Sedative oils for use in bath or massage include **benzoin, bergamot, chamomile, cedar, clary sage, frankincense, geranium, jasmine, lavender, marjoram, melissa, neroli, patchouli, rose, sandalwood,** and **ylang-ylang.** One or more of these oils can be blended with jojoba oil, in a ratio of 30 drops essence to ½ ounce jojoba, to create a personal anxiety-reducing perfume.

ASTHMA

Asthma is one of four fast-growing diseases not yet cured by conventional medicine that have been targeted for study by the new National Institutes of Health Office of Alternative and Complementary Medicine (the other diseases are AIDS, cancer, and heart disease). According to figures compiled by the National Institutes for Health, the ranks of asthma sufferers in this country increased 74 percent in the ten-year period between 1984 and 1994, for a total of about fifteen million American asthmatics. In the same period, fatal asthma attacks grew 59 percent. Children, especially those who live in cities, account for much of the increase, being 50 percent more likely than adults to contract the potentially life-threatening condition.

The likelihood of children developing asthma has been linked to poor diet and overuse of antibiotics. Natural practitioners suggest that asthmatics avoid foods such as dairy products, caffeine, cold drinks, red meat, sugar, and tobacco. Beneficial supplements include vitamin A for tissue repair and immune enhancement; B complex, particularly B5 to reduce stress, B6 and B12 to stimulate the immune system; buffered vitamin C for its antibronchiospastic effect; natural vitamin E, an antioxidant, protects cells from free-radical damage; wheat grass juice; essential fatty acids such as Omega-3, which is anti-inflammatory, found in flaxseed and fish oils; magnesium, to reduce bronchial constriction; and selenium, one of ten essential trace minerals, which works with vitamin E to stop free-radical damage.

Important: All of the following suggestions are meant to complement professional medical care for this potentially life-threatening condition, not to replace it. Always consult with your physician before undertaking complementary remedies for medical conditions.

Herbs: Angelica (**Angelica sinensis** or dong quai), used by Chinese herbalists to prevent and relieve allergic symptoms, as tea or tincture; **astralagus,** to strengthen the lungs and increase the body's ability to protect itself (do not use astralagus if fever or infection are present); **capsicum,** to desensitize airway mucosa to irritants, used as tincture; Chinese **skullcap,** anti-inflammatory, antioxidant, as tea or tincture; **ephedra,** a bronchiodilator, as tea (do not use with children under twelve years of age); **garlic, ginger, goldenseal,** all natural antibiotics; **licorice,** anti-inflammatory, anti-allergy, helps to prevent some of the side effects of cortisone, used as tea or tincture (if using for the long term, be sure to eat lots of potassium-rich foods, such as brewer's yeast, dates, bananas, watercress, and kelp); **lobelia,** antispasmodic, expectorant, promotes release of adrenal hormones that help relax bronchial muscles, as tea or tincture, alone or combined with skunk cabbage or cayenne; **marshmallow,** to soothe bronchial tubes; **mullein,** antispasmodic and bronchial decongestant; **skunk cabbage,** expectorant and respiratory sedative, as tea or tincture, with lobelia and capsicum during acute asthma attacks; **slippery elm,** soothing for mucous membranes; **thyme,** antispasmodic, antibacterial; **turmeric,** has a bronchodilatory effect and can be mixed with a glass of warm water and sipped during an attack; **motherwort** and **skullcap,** to help relieve anxiety.

Homeopathics: Aconite, for sudden onset of attack, may be accompanied by pressure on left side of chest, grasping at throat, and be worse at night or after midnight; **Antimonium tartaricum,** for drowsiness, weakness, heavy perspiration, feeling of suffocation, rattling mucus in bronchial tubes; **Apis,** for asthma that is worse in heat and in the afternoon, accompanied by dislike of being touched and a feeling of being unable to take another breath; **Arsenicum,** for asthma attacks accompanied by exhaustion, restlessness, worse after midnight and when lying on back, shooting pain in upper right lung; **Belladonna,** for a person who feels hot, dry, with uneven breathing, worse at night; **Carbo veg,** for asthma in frail, elderly folks with bluish cast to skin; **Calcarea carbonica,** for symptoms that are worse in the morning, or accompanied by ear infection; **Nux vomica,** asthma attacks on a full stomach or in the morning; **Pothoas,** seasonal asthma; **Sulfur,** asthma accompanied by hot flashes, burning sensation, or sinking of stomach at 11 A.M.

Flower Essences: Agrimony; Rock Rose, for the panic and terror that can accompany a severe asthma attack; **Five Flower** or **Rescue Remedy.**

Essential Oils: Regular aromatic massage of the chest and back can be very beneficial for asthma sufferers. Useful essences include **bergamot** and **lavender,** antispasmodics; **chamomile, clary sage, eucalyptus,** or **frankincense** can also be used in inhalations to promote deep and relaxed breathing; **neroli** and **rose.**

ATHLETE'S FOOT

This uncomfortable condition can be caused by a variety of molds and fungi capable of infecting the outer layers of the skin of the feet, as well as the groin area in hot, humid climates. Keep affected areas dry and clean.

Herbs: Black walnut, extract used externally as a wash, or take capsules internally; **calendula,** antifungal and soothing, use an infusion externally as a wash, or use the oil or ointment to soothe cracked skin; **echinacea,** antifungal, internally as tea or decoction, externally as wash; **garlic,** fresh crushed, applied daily as a poultice, or take internally in capsules; **myrrh,** in a warm water wash and soak.

Homeopathics: Phosphorus, especially with burning, cracking, and bleeding of skin; **Sepia.**

Flower Essences: Crab Apple, for any feelings of uncleanness.

Essential Oils: Lavender, myrrh, tea tree, diluted in alcohol and swabbed on until moisture dries up, then in 3 to 5 percent dilution in oil or cream to heal cracked skin; **thyme** in a foot bath or diluted in oil.

BEDWETTING (ENURESIS)

Occasional bedwetting, up to the age of six, can be chalked up to developmental inevitability as a child learns to control bodily functions. Later bedwetting can be related to emotional problems, allergies, urinary tract infections, spinal problems, or kidney trouble. If bedwetting becomes chronic, consult with your physician to rule out physical abnormalities or disease. To minimize the chances of bedwetting, have the child eat fruit instead of drinking in the evening and stay away from sweets at night. Harsh or punitive parenting can also lead to bedwetting. It's no fun getting up in the middle of the night to change sheets, but parental anger and punishment only make the problem worse. Use a plastic or rubber pad to protect the mattress, and factor in a heavy dose of patience to protect your parent/child bond.

Herbs: Teas, in the early evening, of **cornsilk, cinnamon, fennel, hops, oatstraw,** or **marjoram.**

Homeopathics: Argentum nitricum, when bedwetting is accompanied by poor coordination, craving for sweets, trembling, aversion to heat; **Causticum,** for wetting shortly after going to sleep or during cold or rainy weather; **Equisetum,** when wetting occurs while dreaming; **Kreosotum,** the child urinates in dreams, wets in early part of night, and is hard to awaken; **Pulsatilla,** child may sleep with hands above the head, or urine may have offensive odor; **Sepia,** for brunettes who wet the bed shortly after going to sleep; **Sulfur,** for a child who urinates frequently in the daytime, wets at night, and whose urinary opening may be red and sore.

Flower Essences: If fear is involved, **Mimulus** for known fears; **Aspen** for fears of unknown origin; **Crab Apple** for any lingering feelings of uncleanness.

Essential Oils: Essences that have a healing or strengthening effect on the urinary system include **bergamot, chamomile, eucalyptus, juniper, sandalwood,** and **tea tree,** used in compresses over the lower abdomen.

BITES AND STINGS

The faster a bite or sting is treated, the better the likelihood of reducing pain and inflammation. The acidity of bee stings can be neutralized with an alkaline paste of baking soda. Wasp stings are alkaline, so apply an acidic wash of vinegar or lemon juice. Be sure to remove the stinger. Crushed charcoal tablets can be applied to bee or wasp stings. A paste made of clay can also help draw out poisons. Vitamin B1 supplements, a low-sugar diet, eating garlic and onions, and wearing light-colored clothing may help keep insects away so they don't bite in the first place. Get medical attention if there is an extreme reaction or if the bite is from a poisonous insect such as a black widow or a brown recluse spider.

Herbs: Herbs to try externally as a wash or in a compress are **aloe vera, echinacea, comfrey, lobelia,** and **witch hazel.**

Homeopathics: Apis mellifica, for anything resembling bee sting, wasp or yellow jacket stings, black widow bites, and also for allergic reactions to bee stings; **Arsenicum,** for itching, burning insect stings; **Crotalus horridus,** for insect stings that produce weepiness, talkativeness, or impatience; **Echinacea,** for inflamed insect bites, snake bites, accompanied by chills, nausea, depression, confusion; **Hypericum,** for damaged nerves resulting from animal bites; **Ledum,** for mosquito, snake, or spider bites; **Apis** and **Ledum** together at 30c potency, every fifteen minutes, for venomous bites of unknown origin.

Flower Essences: Five Flower or **Rescue Remedy** can be applied directly to the bite or sting, in liquid or cream form.

Essential Oils: For mosquito bites, **lavender** and **blue chamomile** alone or in combination; **lavender** and **tea tree** help soothe most bites; for flea bites, a tiny bit of **peppermint** can take away the itching, with tea tree added to heal areas already scratched open; **basil, lemon, sage,** or **thyme** in dilution.

BLEEDING

Bleeding is the body's way of washing out debris and invaders when the integrity of the skin, or venal or arterial walls has been broken. If possible, wash the injured area with soap and water, and apply pressure with a cloth or bandage. If bleeding is severe or the result of a serious cut or injury, seek immediate medical attention.

Herbs: Calendula infusion or tincture as first aid, ointment or cream as antiseptic; **cayenne,** to stop bleeding fast, sprinkle cayenne powder or tincture directly on cuts or wounds; **witch hazel** (*Hamamelis*) is an excellent first-aid remedy to stop bleeding; fresh **lemon** juice can also be applied to a wound to stop bleeding, or held in the mouth (not sloshed around) to stop the bleeding that may result after tooth extraction, or when a child loses baby teeth; powdered **sage** can also be sprinkled directly on a cut or scrape to stop bleeding and assist in formation of a scab.

Homeopathics: Arnica, 30c potency up to four times every fifteen minutes, or single dose of 1m potency as first aid for bleeding after injury, surgery, or childbirth.

Flower Essences: The sight of blood frightens many children (and adults!), so try a quick dose of **Five Flower** or **Rescue Remedy** to restore calm.

Essential Oils: A few drops of **lemon, geranium,** and **rose** can be put in a bowl of sterile water, into which a gauze compress can be dipped and then applied with firm pressure against a wound to help stop bleeding; add **lavender** as an antiseptic; **cypress,** in bath or massage, can help slow excessive menstrual bleeding. **See also:** NOSEBLEEDS

BRUISES

Bruises should be treated immediately for best results. Vitamin C with bioflavonoids can be taken as a supplement to strengthen capillary walls in those who bruise easily.

Herbs: Leaves of the **elder tree** applied externally as a poultice; **black walnut, comfrey,** or **aloe vera** externally in a warm poultice; **alfalfa** internally to speed healing.

Homeopathics: Arnica, tincture or ointment externally, pellets internally, for bruises to muscles and soft tissues; **Hypericum,** for bruising that may also involve crushed nerves, or smashed fingers or toes; **Rhus tox,** for bruising as a result of sprains, torn ligaments, pulled tendons; **Ruta graveolens,** especially for bruises accompanied by sprains; **Symphytum,** for bruises to bones.

Flower Essences: Five Flower or **Rescue Remedy** for shock or trauma of injury.

Essential Oils: Apply **Fennel, helichrysm, hyssop, sage**, or **lavender** in a cold compress immediately on injury; **rosemary**, to speed circulation during later stages of healing. I have also used undiluted **lavender** directly on an area immediately after an injury, and have seen the swelling and inflammation actually go down as I watched, with little or no subsequent bruising!

BURNS

Sunburns and scalds from steam, hot water, or beverages are usually first-degree burns that can be treated at home, although if there is any doubt, consult your physician. Sunburns can progress to second-degree burns, which can also be caused by contact with flames or hot metal. Third- and fourth-degree burns can be fatal and must receive prompt medical attention. If blistering occurs, leave the blisters intact to prevent infection.

Herbs: For sunburns or mild burns, wash with **cucumber** juice to soothe; mix 1 tablespoon of almond or safflower oil with the fresh inner pulp of an **aloe vera** leaf and several drops of **lavender** essential oil and apply immediately to a sunburn; **herbal honey** can be applied externally to speed healing and prevent infection, or **comfrey** can be mixed with wheatgerm oil and honey for external application; a poultice of **slippery elm** speeds healing and draws out toxins; **goldenseal** can be used internally and externally to prevent infection.

Homeopathics: Arnica, for shock; **Arsenicum; Cantharis**, especially for burns that blister, burn, or itch; **Causticum**, for painful burns that are slow to heal or if **Cantharis** doesn't help; **Phosphorus**, for electrical burns, after Arnica has been given; **Urtica urens**, for painful, red burns that may itch violently.

Flower Essences: Five Flower or **Rescue Remedy**, for trauma.

Essential Oils: If **lavender** essence can be applied immediately, undiluted, after burning, severity can be greatly reduced and blistering and scarring practically eliminated. If there is no lavender on hand, **chamomile, eucalyptus, niaouli, rosemary,** or **sage** could be used.

Chicken Pox

Kids usually get chicken pox between the ages of five and ten years old, which is good, because this relatively minor childhood disease causes more severe suffering in adults. The virus that causes it, varicella-zoster, can be caught through the air or through physical contact and takes about two weeks to incubate. Initial symptoms may include irritability and sneezing or runny nose. Small red spots then appear on the chest, arms, or face, with blistered centers, and they are very itchy. Scratching breaks open the lesions but doesn't stop the itching. Chicken pox continues to be contagious until about two weeks after the lesions have scabbed over. Try to prevent scratching to minimize scarring and infection. Very young children can have cotton bags or gloves put on their hands. Do not use aspirin, to avoid the possibility of Reye's syndrome, a life-threatening illness characterized by rapid, shallow breathing and vomiting. Oatmeal baths or baths with baking soda and apple cider vinegar can help soothe skin and reduce itching.

Herbs: To bring out eruptions, try a warm bath with infusions of **burdock** and **goldenseal; chamomile** in the bath to soothe the skin and reduce itching, and as a tea to aid sleep and relaxation; **catnip** tea for calming; **aloe vera** or salves of **comfrey** or **goldenseal** to promote healing of lesions; **lemon juice, lime juice,** or **red clover** to purify the blood.

Homeopathics: Aconite, for a child who is apprehensive, feverish, and thirsty, in the early stages before eruptions; **Antimonium crudum,** for chicken pox accompanied by white-coated tongue, irritability, and sores that itch more after a bath; **Arsenicum,** for burning pains and chills; **Belladonna,** for high fever, headache, red face, hot skin, and inability to sleep; **Mercurius,** if there is odorous perspiration and possibly swollen glands; **Rhus tox,** the most commonly used homeopathic remedy, after eruptions have come up and until they're gone, if the eruptions turn into open sores, and if symptoms are much worse at night; **Variolinum,** after being exposed but before symptoms appear.

Flower Essences: Children's emotional states when they're ill can vary widely. Read through the descriptions at the end of Chapter 4 to determine which apply to your child.

Essential Oils: Tea tree is the aromatherapist's first choice, in a tepid bath, alone or with **chamomile,** to reduce itching and promote healing; try **bergamot** or **eucalyptus** in the bath on first news of exposure; or make a spray of **rose water** with a few drops of **tea tree, chamomile or lavender,** and shake and spritz on eruptions.

COLDS: see RESPIRATORY PROBLEMS

COLD SORES AND CANKER SORES

Cold sores and fever blisters are caused by the herpes simplex virus, and they can be aggravated by a cold or flu, stress, or exposure to intense sunlight. Canker sores are not caused by herpes simplex and generally appear inside the mouth as a result of allergies or low immune function. **Borax,** diluted in water, can be used as a mouthwash to soothe canker sores. **Lysine,** an amino acid, can be helpful in reducing the severity of herpes outbreaks when taken as a supplement. Vitamins C, A, and E, and zinc help bolster resistance. Avoid acidic foods, meat, poultry, nuts, and chocolate.

Herbs: Bayberry tree bark, infused, as a mouthwash; tincture of **calendula, goldenseal, St. John's Wort,** and **myrrh,** singly or in combination, can be applied to sores.

Homeopathics: Dulcamara, for lesions that appear accompanied by swollen glands, with a cold, or in cold, damp weather; **Hepar sulph,** for extremely painful lesions, possibly with pus, accompanied by irritability; **Mercurius,** sores with drooling and high fever; **Natrum mur,** at first symptoms of sensitivity or tingling, with dry lips, thirst, white blisters on lips or gums; **Rhus tox,** dry, cracked lips, insomnia, especially if Natrum mur has not worked.

Flower Essences: Five Flower or **Rescue Remedy** can be applied directly to sores.

Essential Oils: Lavender or **tea tree** can be dabbed onto sores; or try a 1:2 part blend of rose and melissa.

COLIC

Colic is acute abdominal pain, often accompanied by gas or gurgling in the stomach, that occurs in babies under four months of age, usually about the same time each night, lasting for several patience-trying, nerve-shattering hours. Colic can result from a baby's allergies or sensitivities to foods eaten by a nursing mother, such as acidic foods, wheat, dairy, chocolate, or coffee. Most babies grow out of colic by the age of three or four months. If crying persists for more than three hours, or if the baby's cries are piercing or anguished or accompanied by other symptoms of illness, call your physician. Try daily infant massage and carrying the baby in a front pack during the day to increase relaxation and calmness.

Herbs: A teaspoon at a time of weak, tepid tea made with **chamomile, dill seed, fennel seed,** or **mint; ginger** and **clove** can also help relieve gas.

Homeopathics: Aconite, when symptoms are not relieved by any position; **Colocynthis,** when baby is anxious, doubles up with pain, may have diarrhea; **Carbo veg,** when baby is pale, upper abdomen is bloated, and legs and feet are cold; **Chamomilla,** colic and a baby that may also be teething, that screams and wants to be held or carried constantly; **Lycopodium,** when lower abdomen is swollen, baby may wake up at 4 A.M.; **Magnesia phos,** when warmth and pressure may help to pass gas and baby tends to draw up knees into fetal position; **Nux vomica,** when baby is cold and irritable, strains unsuccessfully to have bowel movement, may be aggravated by mother drinking alcohol, eating spicy foods; **Pulsatilla,** for colic with gurgling in the stomach, bloating, and after breast-feeding mother eats ice cream, fatty foods, or fruit.

Flower Essences: Five Flower or **Rescue Remedy** can be applied topically.

Essential Oils: A drop of **chamomile, mandarin, melissa,** or **tangerine** can be added to a base oil of sweet almond or sesame oil for gentle massage of the lower abdomen and lower back.

CONJUNCTIVITIS

Inflammation of the conjunctiva, which is the mucous membrane that covers the eyeball and lines the eyelids, causes the eye to look bloodshot. When it accompanies a cold, there may be a clear discharge. It can also be caused by an irritant lodged in the eye, in which case an eyewash and some rest will solve the problem. If caused by an allergy, there will be itching. Infection by a bacteria or virus may cause a thick, greenish yellow discharge that crusts the eye shut during sleep. Bacterial conjunctivitis is contagious, and hands, bedclothes, or utensils such as eyecups should be washed immediately after touching the infected eye. Grated apple or potato can be used as poultices, and a drop of lemon juice in a glass of water can be used as an external cleanser. If the condition doesn't clear up within a few days, or grows worse, consult a physician.

Herbs: Internally, **echinacea, elder flower, eyebright, goldenseal**, and **sage**; externally, try compresses soaked in infusions of **chamomile, elder flower, eyebright, goldenseal**, or **calendula**.

Homeopathics: Apis mel, for burning, puffy lids that stick together and feel better from cold compresses; **Argentum nitricum,** when the whites of the eyes and the corners are red and sensitive to light and warmth, but better in cold air; **Euphrasia,** for itching, inflamed eyes with burning tears, constantly watering eyes, headache, and runny nose; **Natrum mur,** for swollen lids, burning tears, eyes may feel bruised, mucus or pus discharge; **Pulsatilla,** conjunctivitis with cold or measles, with thick, yellow discharge that aggravates itching and styes on lower lids, and symptoms worse in the morning; **Sulfur,** for extreme sensitivity to light, bloodshot, painful, itchy eyes, hot tears.

Essential Oils: Essential oils are, as a rule, too irritating to use in eyes and mucous membranes. Floral waters or hydrolates from the distillation process should be used instead. Cotton pads can be soaked in **rose water** or **hydrosols of rose** or **chamomile** and applied to the eyes to soothe and disinfect.

CONSTIPATION: see GASTROINTESTINAL PROBLEMS

CUTS AND SCRAPES

Deep or long cuts may require emergency medical attention. Minor cuts and scrapes should first be cleansed of dirt and washed with an antiseptic infusion.

Herbs: Wash with an antiseptic infusion of **echinacea,** which can also be taken internally as tea or capsules to reduce pus formation and speed healing; diluted **lemon** juice or **calendula** tincture can also be used to cleanse, but do not use calendula over time on a deep wound as it may encourage superficial healing while the wound is still open underneath; powdered **sage** or **cayenne** or cayenne tincture can be put over the wound to stop bleeding and help formation of a scab; **garlic,** a natural antibiotic, can be crushed into a paste and spread over the wound, then washed off after fifteen to thirty minutes (leaving it on longer might burn the skin); **papaya** can also be mashed and thinly applied several times a day to promote external tissue repair; **aloe vera** can be applied externally to prevent scarring and improve healing; **goldenseal** prevents infection and speeds healing.

Homeopathics: Arnica, if there is bruising or shock to the body; **Hepar sulph,** three times daily to promote healing; **Hypericum ointment,** if the scrape is very painful, or tincture for deep or infected cuts, or pellets if there are shooting pains; **Ledum,** if the injury is a result of puncture with a sharp instrument.

Flower Essences: Five Flower or **Rescue Remedy** to soothe the trauma of injury.

Essential Oils: Cleanse wound with water to which a few drops of **lavender, eucalyptus, lemon, niaouli,** and/or **tea tree** have been added. The same essential oils can be used in compresses to promote healing and reduce the risk of infection. A drop or two of **lavender** applied undiluted to the gauze or bandage (such as Band-Aid brand) placed over a cut or scrape works as a natural antibiotic and promotes tissue repair.
See also: BLEEDING

DEPRESSION

Mild depression may sometimes accompany the changes or stresses of life and takes a variety of forms, from restlessness and insomnia to lethargy and sleeping late. If depression deepens, continues for a protracted period, or adversely affects one's ability to function, professional help should be sought.

Herbs: Antidepressant and nervine herbs include **borage, cayenne, lime blossom/linden tree flower/tilia tea, oats, rosemary, skullcap, valerian,** and **vervain,** to be taken in the form of tincture or tea; **St. John's Wort** extract.

Homeopathics: Aesculus hippocastanum, for irritable depression, possibly with frontal headache and back or body aches, chills in late afternoon, fever at night, worse in the morning and from walking, better in cool, open air; **Agnus castus,** for sad depression, fear of death, possibly with dilated pupils and itchy eyes, impotence, and/or lack of desire; **Apis mel,** for depression accompanied by weepiness, irritability, sadness, suspicion, or jealousy; **Conium,** for mental depression following overexcitement, no interest in anything, worse from lying down, may be PMS-related; **Gelsemium,** for listlessness, apathy, wanting to be left alone; **Helonias,** for profound melancholy, better from keeping the mind busy, possibly accompanied by lower backache and heavy or too frequent menses, tendency to uterine prolapse; **Ignatia,** for depression with moodiness, sighing, and sobbing, possibly as a result of a shock or disappointment, worse in the morning and from smoking or drinking coffee, better from eating; **Lycopodium,** for melancholy, especially on awakening in the morning, with right-sided symptoms that are worse between 4 P.M. and 8 P.M.; **Nux vomica,** for sullen, fault-finding depression, ugly mood, great sensitivity to smells, noises, and light, worse in the morning and from tobacco, alcohol, coffee, or open air, better after a nap; **Pulsatilla,** for weepy depression that loves sympathy; **Sepia,** for lifeless depression accompanied by moodiness and lack of interest in loved ones, being easily offended and with a tendency to be mean.

Flower Essences: Aspen, for depression accompanied by vague feelings of dread; **Cherry Plum,** for depression accompanied by a fear of having a breakdown or thoughts of violence to oneself or others; **Clematis,** for depression that feels like sleepwalking or moving through a fog; **Elm,** for depression as a result of being overwhelmed; **Gentian,** for depression accompanied by self-doubt or discouragement at the slightest obstacle; **Gorse,** for hopelessness; **Honeysuckle,** for lack of interest in the present or future because of preoccupation with the past, especially happier times; **Hornbeam,** for depression accompanied by a feeling that one is not strong enough mentally or physically to deal with life's challenges; **Larch,** for depression with low self-confidence and feelings of failure; **Mustard,** for sudden bouts of inexplicable gloom; **Oak,** for depression with a fighting spirit in the face of all odds; **Olive,** for depression accompanied by exhaustion or fatigue, when life seems to be just too much of a struggle; **Pine,** for those who blame themselves for everything; **Star of Bethlehem,** for depression following a shock, accident, or loss; **Sweet Chestnut,** for anguish that feels unbearable, and when the future appears hopeless; **White Chestnut,** for depression accompanied by obsessive thinking; **Wild Oat,** for depression as a result of not knowing one's path or calling in life; **Wild Rose,** for depression that takes the form of resignation or giving up; **Willow,** for depression accompanied by resentment over a setback in life.

Essential Oils: Chamomile, clary sage, lavender, sandalwood, and **ylang-ylang** have a sedative effect while elevating mood; **bergamot, geranium, melissa,** and **rose** elevate mood for those who don't want or need the sedative effect; **neroli** and **jasmine** for depression accompanied by anxiety; in bath, massage, or as personal perfume; **marjoram** for depression caused by grief; **cypress, sage,** and **thyme** for balancing the nervous system; the sunny aromas of citruses such as **grapefruit, lemon, orange,** and **tangerine** for promoting cheerfulness.
See also: ANXIETY and STRESS

DIAPER RASH

Diaper rash can be caused by a number of things, including soaps, lotions, or powders used on the baby's skin, detergents used to wash the diapers, fungal or bacterial infection, or an allergic reaction to something eaten by the baby or breast-feeding mother. Disposable diapers, plastic pants, artificial fragrances, or alcohol in baby wipes, creams, or laundry soaps should be avoided. Change diapers frequently, and allow the baby to go without a diaper as much as possible. A bright red, raised rash with definite borders that extends from the area of the anus or occurs in folds of skin may be caused by yeast and may be soothed with a poultice of acidophilus or yogurt. The breast-feeding mother can also take supplements of acidophilus, and may want to avoid potentially allergenic or yeast-aggravating foods such as dairy products or foods containing yeast, sugar, or caffeine. If acidic urine is causing the problem, 1 tablespoon of baking soda in $\frac{1}{2}$ cup of water can be used to wash the baby's bottom, to increase alkalinity. Vitamin E can be applied to the rash to soothe and promote healing, or plain cornstarch can be used as a baby powder to keep skin dry. If the rash worsens or won't go away, consult your physician.

Herbs: An infusion of **bay leaves** can be used as a wash for a yeast-caused rash; **calendula** lotion, **aloe vera, goldenseal,** or **comfrey** ointment may soothe rashes caused by irritation or bacteria; **calendula** infusion can be used in the bath; **evening primrose** extract or lotion can be used to reduce inflammation and promote healing.

Homeopathics: Calcarea carb for chronic diaper rash in babies who are fat or flabby, with large, round heads, runny noses, cold feet, and an allergy or aversion to milk; **Sulfur,** for chronic diaper rash in hot, active, messy babies who may have a tendency to spit and have redness of lips and other orifices.

Flower Essences: Agrimony, for diaper rash that may result from inner emotional turbulence in a baby who, on the outside, is always cheerful and smiling.

Essential Oils: A drop of **lavender** or **chamomile** diluted in oil or milk can be added to the bath to prevent bacterial infection; **tea tree** in bath or ointment for fungal infections; diapers can be rinsed in water containing **lavender** or **tea tree; rose water** can be used to soothe and disinfect skin when changing diapers.

DIARRHEA: see GASTROINTESTINAL PROBLEMS

Earache

There are several medical terms for ear infections, the most common of which is otitis media, affecting the middle ear. Otitis externa involves the outer ear; otitis interna, the inner ear. Often an earache occurs as a secondary infection from bacteria proliferating during a cold or sinusitis. In very young children, an ear infection may be indicated by behaviors such as pulling at their ears, moving their heads in strange ways, crying, and not wanting to lie down.

Because infection can spread through the eustachian tubes fairly rapidly, ear infections are potentially dangerous and should never be ignored. If symptoms don't improve within twenty-four hours, or if there is a high fever, consult your physician.

Antibiotics are routinely prescribed for ear infections to prevent possible scarring that might impair hearing. However, there is evidence to indicate that it may be healthier in all but the most severe cases to allow the body to fight the infection, since overuse of antibiotics is associated with recurring ear infections and later immune response problems as well as ADD/ADHD.

Natural treatments work best if begun immediately, on onset of symptoms, and they can often be continued even if antibiotics are prescribed. During an ear infection, keep the child calm and quiet. Avoid cow's milk and dairy products, and give extra vitamin E, C, and B complex. If antibiotics are given, watch for allergic reactions in the form of rashes, swelling, or difficult breathing. Use acidophilus supplements for a month after such treatment to restore the healthy flora in the digestive system.

Herbs: Garlic or the heart of an **onion** can be boiled, cooled, and applied to the outside of the ear as a poultice; **garlic** or **mullein** oil can be put on a cotton ball and placed in the ear, and garlic capsules can be taken to bolster overall health; a cotton bag filled with salt can be heated in a pan until warmed and used as a compress; **lobelia, hops, St. John's Wort** in tea or tincture for calming and reducing inflammation; **echinacea** and/or **goldenseal** if ear problems are chronic or if there is a discharge from the ear; **passionflower** for calming; plantain tincture, **St. John's Wort oil,** or **witch hazel** externally to reduce inflammation and pain.

Homeopathics: Aconite, for sudden, throbbing pain after being out in cold or windy weather, child is anxious, feels worse at night; **Belladonna,** when ear is red inside and out, pain comes on suddenly, after a draft, piercing pain, possibly worse in the right ear, may be accompanied by high fever and sore throat or swollen glands. Belladonna is an onset remedy, not used after the first day or two; **Chamomilla,** when pain is unbearable, child is irritable and wants to be carried, one or both cheeks are red, worse from heat or wind; **Ferrum phos,** for use at the onset of any earache, especially if earache is on the left side, outer ear is pink, child is tired; **Hepar sulph,** for otitis media, when infection has progressed, worse from touch, child is overly sensitive, prone to tantrums, may have dry cough; **Lycopodium,** when earache is worse on right side, or starts there and moves left, worse between 4:00 P.M. and 8:00 P.M., especially in children who hide their insecurities by boasting or bullying behavior; **Mercurius,** commonly used for chronic ear infections, especially with discharge that is worse at night, possibly accompanied by swollen glands, sore throat, and bad breath, better after blowing the nose, worse from hot or cold applications; **Mercurius iodatus flavus,** for right-sided earaches; **M. iodatus ruber,** for left-sided earaches; **Plantago,** for earache that accompanies teething, tincture can be rubbed onto the gums; **Pulsatilla,** when ear is swollen and hot and may itch inside, and for recurrent ear infections in a child who is mild-tempered and weepy, worse from warmth, better in fresh air.

Flower Essences: Five Flower or **Rescue Remedy** drops or cream can be applied to the outside of the ear.

Essential Oils: Lavender or **chamomile,** in warm compresses or diluted in oil for gentle massage around the outer part of the ear, are the classic aromatherapy remedies; **clary sage,** diluted in warm oil and massaged gently around the outside of the ear, can have an amazing effect on reducing pain; a few drops of **lavender** can also be placed on a cotton ball that can then be inserted into the ear as an antibacterial. Frequent ear infections indicate a need for systemic cleansing and building of resistance through improved diet and daily fortifying baths and massage with immune-building essences such as **eucalyptus, lavender, niaouli, tea tree,** and **thyme.**

Fever

Fever can be a reaction to illness or, especially in children, can come on the heels of intense or repressed emotions such as fear or anger. Because fever is part of the body's response to infection, it should not necessarily be indiscriminately repressed. If, however, a fever in a child rises above 104 degrees F, if the child loses consciousness, starts to twitch or convulse, or is hot on one side and cold on the other, call your physician immediately.

Herbs: Catnip or peppermint tea is cooling; elder flower, lime flower to help break a fever; for fevers with chest congestion, hyssop or elecampane; for fever after a fright, motherwort or passionflower; ginger and alfalfa to strengthen the system overall; goldenseal or elecampane if there is mucus; yarrow tea or tincture (children over five only).

Homeopathics: Aconite, at onset of dry fever that comes on suddenly after a chill or a fright, child may be thirsty, flushed, or alternately flushed and pale; Arsenicum, for fever with chills and restlessness, worse between 12 A.M. and 3 A.M.; Belladonna, for sudden high fever with red lips and flushed cheeks, dry heat radiating from face or head and cold feet or hands, fever worst at night; Ferrum phos, at the beginning stage of fever and symptoms with slow onset; Nux vomica, for fever after overeating, loss of sleep, or as a side effect of a drug; Pulsatilla, for fever with chills, no thirst; Sulfur, for fever with phlegm and reddened skin, diarrhea on waking, thirsty with foul-smelling sweat.

Flower Essences: Five Flower or Rescue Remedy, especially for fevers brought on by fear, shock, or strong emotions.

Essential Oils: Bergamot, chamomile, eucalyptus, lavender, and/or peppermint in tepid water for sponging down or compresses applied to the feet or head; basil, chamomile, cypress, juniper, lavender, rosemary, tea tree, in bath or massage to help break a fever and induce sweating; clove, eucalyptus, lemon, and/or sage essences in a room spray to disinfect atmosphere.

Food Poisoning: see Gastrointestinal Problems

GASTROINTESTINAL PROBLEMS (Constipation, Diarrhea, Digestive Problems)

Good digestion is integral to good health. The gastrointestinal system is easily influenced by the endocrine and nervous systems, which is why emotional upsets so often manifest as disturbances in digestive or eliminative processes. In the event of diarrhea, be sure to provide plenty of fluids, since young children and babies can become dehydrated very quickly. If symptoms persist for more than a day or two, consult a qualified medical practitioner.

Herbs: Barberry contains an alkaloid called berberine, also found in **goldenseal,** which is effective against intestinal bacteria; **bistort root, astringent,** for diarrhea; **blackberry root** or leaves, **blackberry brandy,** for its astringent effect on diarrhea; **cascara sagrada,** for constipation; **chamomile** *(Matricaria chamomilla),* useful in colic from infants through adults, and also beneficial during bouts of stomach flu, for its antibacterial effect and to reduce inflammation, relieve spasms, and counteract associated flatulence and pain; **fennel,** as tea, to relieve constipation and promote healthy digestion; **garlic,** a potent intestinal antimicrobial, inhibits pathogenic organisms without affecting the beneficial flora and increases bile secretions and decreases spasms, which can help to detoxify the bowels; **ginger,** to improve digestion and alleviate digestive problems, also to alleviate morning sickness during pregnancy; **goldenseal,** an astringent and tonic, benefits the mucous membranes lining the gut wall and can be useful for digestive irritations and diarrhea; **green apple,** peeled, pectin absorbs bacterial toxins; **guava leaves,** astringent and antibacterial, have been used historically to slow the intestines during diarrhea; **peppermint,** as tea, to relieve indigestion; **psyllium seeds,** for constipation; **senna,** to relieve constipation.

Aqua Mirabilis: This medieval "miracle water" can be taken one spoonful daily to improve digestion and ease constipation. If using fresh herbs, double the quantity of herbal material. Put 3 tablespoons each of **angelica, rosemary, marjoram, costmary, hyssop, wormwood, mint, thyme,** and **sage** into 2 quarts of vodka or brandy. Set in the sun for two weeks, then strain and bottle. Can also be used externally on compresses to help heal sores on the skin.

Homeopathics: Abies canadensis, for indigestion caused by overeating, with cravings for meat and pickles, accompanied by chills and possibly night sweats; **Arsenicum,** for food poisoning, burning diarrhea that irritates the anus, worse after midnight and from cold, better from warm drinks or compresses; **Chamomilla,** for nausea caused by too much coffee; **Cocculus,** especially for light-haired females, nausea, morning sickness, motion sickness, possibly with hiccups, yawning, and/or great desire to sing; **Graphites,** for nausea, especially from overconsumption of sweets, stomach pain, bloating, flatulence, constipation with mucus connecting hard stools, chronic, liquid, dark brown diarrhea, worse from warm drinks, at night, during menses, better in the dark and from wrapping up, child may be disobedient and impudent; **Ipecacuanha,** for persistent nausea and vomiting, may be accompanied by irritability and contempt, worse periodically and from lying down; **Mercurius,** for nausea not relieved by vomiting, green, smelly stools in infants, painful defecation, worse in the evening and at night; **Nux vomica,** for diarrhea caused by rich or spicy food, bloating, gas, nausea improved by vomiting, accompanied by irritability; **Sepia,** for nausea in the morning before breakfast, nausea caused by tobacco smoke, vomiting after eating, worse from the sight or smell of food, craving for vinegar and pickles, indigestion with bloating and sour burps, constipation with feeling of a ball in the rectum, infantile diarrhea, worse before noon and in the evening, in cold air, before a thunderstorm, and from milk, better after sleep and from hot applications.

Flower Essences: For digestive disturbances that result from emotional states, refer to complete listing at the end of Chapter 4.

Essential Oils: With clockwise massage over the abdomen for constipation or diarrhea, **marjoram, rosemary,** or **fennel** diluted in a carrier oil base; for diarrhea, antispasmodics such as **chamomile, cypress, eucalyptus, lavender, neroli,** or **peppermint**; for nervous diarrhea, **chamomile, lavender, neroli**; for warming and to improve digestion, **benzoin, black pepper, ginger, fennel**; for diarrhea caused by viral infection, **eucalyptus.**

Headache

Headaches can have a variety of causes, from stress, and fatigue to sinus infections or allergic reaction to food or chemicals. Recurrent headaches may be indicative of more serious problems, and professional help should be sought. Headaches in children can be caused by dehydration. Try giving them a glass of water.

Herbs: Basil and **rosemary,** for headaches following intense mental effort; **lemon balm, chamomile, lavender, passionflower, skullcap,** or **vervain,** to relax and relieve tension; **feverfew,** for migraine headaches; **white willow,** for pain relief; **ginger,** for general symptomatic relief.

Homeopathics: Aconite, for sudden, violent headache, may be centered in forehead or feel as if a band is tightening around the head, accompanied by anxiety and thirst, worse at night; **Belladonna,** for bursting, throbbing pain, usually centered in the forehead or around the eyes, worse from bending forward, lying flat, or moving the eyes, better from sitting up or bending the head back, possibly with dizziness and sensitivity to light; **Bryonia,** for steady, bursting headache, may settle over left eye, any movement makes it worse, comes on in the morning and gets worse throughout the day, may precede development of other symptoms, child is grumpy, refuses sympathy, and wants to be left alone; **Gelsemium,** for headache with weakness and tiredness, can hardly open the eyes, head heavy, aching may start in neck or back of head and spread to forehead, settling over eye or temple, worse in the morning, from heat, and from the sun, better lying down with head raised, may accompany the flu; **Hypericum,** for headache following a blow to the head or spine; **Ignatia,** for emotional headaches, may feel crampy or as if a nail is being driven into the skull, aggravated by talking, tobacco smoke, or strong odors, better after eating; **Nux vomica,** for headache with nausea and aversion to food, worse in the morning and from exertion, lack of sleep, or coughing, migraine or hangover headaches; **Pulsatilla,** for headaches from overeating or indulgence in fatty foods or ice cream, from getting soaked, or related to grief or sadness, worse in the evening, after eating or being in the sun, from coughing or blowing the nose, and better from open air and cold compresses with the head propped up, may happen at school, and frontal headache may be accompanied by digestive difficulties; **Sanguinaria,** for right-sided pain from back of head into eye, worse from sun, better after vomiting, in the dark, or from pressure on head or neck; **Spigelia,** for left-sided pain, deep in eyes, forehead, or temple, accompanied by stiff neck and shoulders, worse from warmth, better from cool applications.

Flower Essences: If the headache has emotional causes, see complete descriptions of flower essences at the end of Chapter 4.

Essential Oils: Lavender and **peppermint** are analgesic oils that can be used alone or in combination, diluted and rubbed on the temples or in cool compresses to the head or neck; **rosemary,** for headache that comes on following mental exertion; **lavender, peppermint, rosemary,** or **eucalyptus** in inhalation for sinus-related headaches; **lavender, melissa,** or **neroli** for nervous tension headaches, which a few minutes of relaxation and deep breathing and aromatic massage to the neck and shoulders can sometimes help to relieve.

HEAD LICE

If you have school-age children, chances are they will be exposed to head lice, especially in preschool and lower grades where they spend a lot of time in close physical contact and sitting or lying on rugs and floors. As children get older, the problem becomes less common, unless they have younger siblings. Once lice are established they can be very difficult and frustrating to get rid of, since even one egg can cause a reinfestation.

Itching and scratching of the head should be investigated immediately in strong light, since the egg cases (nits) that adhere to hair strands are tiny but easier to see in sunlight. After treating, wash and vacuum everything (including your car), and make sure that each family member has a personal hairbrush that is washed and sterilized daily. Wash stuffed animals and/or pop them into the dryer for twenty minutes. Commercial preparations often contain insecticides, which may or may not succeed in killing live lice and nits and generally should not be used as frequently as is sometimes required to fully eradicate the problem. Poor diet and sugar consumption are related to chronic infestation. Useful supplements include vitamin C and bioflavonoids and vitamin A and beta-carotene. A vinegar rinse will help to loosen nits.

Herbs: California bay infusion, as a preventive hair rinse; **echinacea, garlic,** and/or **goldenseal,** to help fight infestation and prevent recurrence.

Homeopathics: Some practitioners believe that recurrent infestation with head lice is indicative of a need for constitutional treatment under the guidance of a professional homeopath.

Flower Essences: Crab Apple, if there are lingering feelings of uncleanness.

Essential Oils: Tea tree can be diluted in an oil carrier and rubbed into the hair, followed by careful, section by section combing with a fine-toothed nit comb. Put a white cloth or T-shirt on the child and wipe the nits from the comb frequently. Live lice can be put into a bowl of water. A combination of **eucalyptus, pennyroyal,** and **rosemary** diluted in an oil base can be used as well. Follow up with several consecutive shampoos to remove all of the oil and daily scalp and hair checks for the next two weeks to remove any remaining nits.

HYPERACTIVITY: see ADD/ADHD

IMMUNE SUPPORT

A strong immune system is necessary for the body to deal success-fully with exposure to viruses, bacteria, and toxins and to heal from illnesses or injuries. Stress or abuse through poor nutrition or bad lifestyle habits can deplete the immune response, opening the way for infection and diseases ranging from allergies to cancer and AIDS. Drugs, even those that seem relatively harmless such as aspirin, antibiotics, and vaccinations, can all weaken the immune system, as can exposure to chemicals and pollutants in the environ-ment. A variety of fresh, raw, organically produced foods and whole grains help to keep a child's (and an adult's) system healthy. Immune-boosting supplements include vitamin A and beta-carotene, vitamins C, E, and B complex, and the minerals selenium and zinc.

Herbs: Astragalus, goldenseal, and **thyme,** for antibacterial action and overall strengthening; **echinacea,** a natural antibiotic, stimulates immune function, though it should be taken only for limited periods; **capsicum** or **cayenne** boosts circulation; **garlic,** a natural antibiotic, helps prevent disease; **ginseng,** an adaptogen; **rose hips** are nourishing and strengthening for the immune system; **fennel** stabilizes the nervous system; **burdock, cleavers,** and **red clover** cleanse the blood; **elder berries, nettles,** and **rosemary** are general tonics.

Homeopathics: Constitutional treatment can improve immune response and should be conducted under the guidance of a licensed homeopath.

Flower Essences: A balanced emotional state helps preserve a healthy immune system. For specifics, see the complete listing at the end of Chapter 4.

Essential Oils: Bergamot, black pepper, cajeput, eucalyptus, geranium, ginger, lemongrass, niaouli, rosemary, or tea tree can be used in aromatic bath, massage, or diffusers to help strengthen the immune response.

INDIGESTION: see Gastrointestinal Problems

INFLUENZA: see RESPIRATORY PROBLEMS and/or GASTROINTESTINAL PROBLEMS

INSOMNIA

Everyone's needs are unique when it comes to sleep. Occasional sleeplessness can be caused by anxiety, excitement, or illness. Meditation, warm baths, gentle massage, and relaxation exercises can help to relax body and mind and alleviate nervous tension in preparation for a good night's rest. Chronic sleep problems or wakefulness accompanied by depression may require professional evaluation and treatment.

Herbs: Borage, chamomile, hops, kava kava root, lemon balm, lime flowers, orange blossom, passionflower, skullcap,

valerian, or **vervain,** in tincture or infusion, in bedtime bath or tea.

Homeopathics: Aconite, for insomnia accompanied by anxious dreams, restlessness; **Anacardium,** for sleepless episodes that go on for several nights, possibly with anxiety-filled dreams; **Chamomilla,** for moaning or crying in sleep, eyes may be partially open, anxious dreams; **Coca,** when sleepy but nervous and unable to rest, also night wakefulness due to teething; **Coffea,** for insomnia from overexcitement, mental activity, or teething pain, especially waking at 3 A.M.; **Passiflora,** for exhaustion or stress resulting in insomnia, also for infants and elderly people; **Pulsatilla,** when sleepy in the afternoon, then wide awake at night, waking unrefreshed, may sleep with hands above head; **Scutellaria,** for sudden waking, sleeplessness due to nerves.

Flower Essences: Aspen, for wakefulness caused by apprehension or dread; **Chicory,** for insomnia due to worry over loved ones; **Mimulus,** for insomnia caused by fear; **White Chestnut,** for an overactive mind full of repetitive or unwanted thoughts.

Essential Oils: Chamomile (especially Roman), **lavender, marjoram,** or **neroli,** in a bedtime bath or massage, or on a cotton ball or tissue placed in the pillowcase.
See also: ANXIETY

MEASLES

Early symptoms of this common childhood disease resemble oncoming cold symptoms: sore throat, red eyes, cough, feverishness. There may be small white spots inside the cheeks. Several days later an itchy rash will appear on the neck and behind the ears, progressing downward to the rest of the body. Like chicken pox, the disease is most contagious in the few days before the spots appear. Keep the child in bed and sponge him or her down to soothe itching and feverishness. German measles are milder than regular measles but pose a threat to a pregnant woman because they can cause birth defects in the fetus during the first trimester. In rare cases, encephalitis occurs as a complication of measles. Be on the lookout for excessive drowsiness and extreme headache or irritability, and call your physician for advice if you observe these symptoms.

Herbs: Boneset, burdock, chamomile, or **elder flower** infusions to soothe, promote healing, and bring down fever; **calendula, chamomile, chickweed,** or **marshmallow** infusion can be sponged on the rash to relieve itching.

Homeopathics: Aconite, at the first stage, with fever, dry cough, restless anxiety, skin burning or itching, tossing and turning in bed; **Belladonna,** at the first stage, with sudden onset of fever, flushed face, throbbing headache, no thirst, difficulty sleeping; **Bryonia,** when the eruptions are slow to come out; **Euphrasia,** in the first stage with pronounced eye symptoms, fever and rash, sensitivity to light, daytime cough; **Ferrum phos,** in early stages if Aconite doesn't help; **Pulsatilla,** mild or later cases, after fever has subsided, possibly accompanied by earache, dry cough at night, runny nose, lack of thirst, also for eye problems following the illness; **Rhus tox,** for intensely itchy rash, worse at night and while resting.

Flower Essences: Chicory, if child is overly whiny and clingy; **Crab Apple,** during recovery for cleansing; **Mimulus** if child is fearful or anxious about being ill.

Essential Oils: Chamomile, eucalyptus, or **lavender** added to tepid water for sponging down; **eucalyptus** on exposure as a preventative.

MUMPS

Mumps is a viral disease, characterized by swelling of the parotid salivary glands, which are below the earlobe in the neck. It is contagious from the day before the symptoms manifest until the swelling of the glands has completely subsided. Acidic beverages and spices should be avoided as they can cause pain in the swollen salivary glands. Encephalitis is a rare complication associated with mumps. (See Measles for symptom list.)

Herbs: Balm, borage, chamomile, echinacea, or **yarrow** as tea to soothe and strengthen.

Homeopathics: Aconite, at early stages, rapid onset, restlessness and thirst, sudden fever, worse from warmth, better in open air; **Belladonna,** the most often used homeopathic treatment, fast and intense onset, red and hot parotid glands, may be accompanied by burning sore throat and shooting pains, and redness of the face; **Bryonia,** for mumps with extreme grumpiness, slightest movement causes pain, dry lips, thirst for cold water; **Mercurius,** when submaxillary glands are also swollen, bad breath, night sweats; **Phytolacca,** when glands are hard, submaxillary glands may also be swollen, swallowing is difficult, skin is pale, worse at night and in cold, wet weather; **Pilocarpinum,** also a popular mumps remedy among homeopaths, for heavy sweating and salivation, thirstiness, general weakness; **Pulsatilla,** for the later stages of mumps, especially when accompanied by whiny, weepy moods, mumps in adults, symptoms worse at night and when lying down; **Rhus tox,** left side is more swollen, chilliness, burning thirst, cold sores, achiness, worse at night, better from movement.

Essential Oils: Chamomile and/or **lavender** in compresses to the neck; **eucalyptus** and **thyme** as a room spray to prevent spreading of infection.

NAUSEA: see GASTROINTESTINAL PROBLEMS

NERVOUSNESS: see ANXIETY

NOSEBLEEDS

Many children experience nosebleeds as a result of damage to capillaries in the nose during colds or allergies when the nose is blown constantly or too hard, from nose picking, or from dry air. Generally, a nosebleed will stop in a few minutes. If it doesn't, have the child lay down on his/her back after blowing the nose to clear out any mucus. Instruct him or her to breathe through the mouth, and pinch the nostrils shut if necessary. Use a vaporizer to humidify dry air. Placing the feet in ice water or putting a cold compress under the neck may also help to stop bleeding. If nosebleeds occur frequently with no apparent cause, or subsequent to a head injury, or if the child is also vomiting, sleepy, or "out of it," call your physician.

Herbs: **Calendula** or **horsetails** infusion or tincture in a compress; **witch hazel (***Hamamelis***)**, excellent first aid to apply to
bleeding of any kind, especially when the blood doesn't immediately clot, acts as an astringent and also soothes, in an infusion or
tincture of leaves or roots; a rolled-up leaf of **wormwood** inserted
into the nostril is a traditional Chinese remedy; **yarrow** infusion
or tincture as wash or compress.

Homeopathics: **Aconite,** for nosebleed accompanied by profuse
menstruation in women, or with great anxiety in children;
Arnica, if as a result of a blow or injury; **Ferrum phos**, especially
when blood is bright red; **Ipecacuanha,** for profuse, spurting, or
frequent nosebleeds; **Lachesis,** when nostrils are sensitive;
Phosphorus, especially for children who grow fast, may be tall
and slim, with a sensitive, alert, artistic temperament;
Phosphoricum acidum, for nosebleeds accompanied by nervous
exhaustion or occurring during or following growth spurts.

Flower Essences: The sight of blood frightens many children,
and **Five Flower** or **Rescue Remedy** can be given externally or
internally to restore calm.

Essential Oils: **Cypress, lemon,** or **terebinth** in compresses.

PARASITES

Parasites are often contracted by children between the ages of two
and five years through contact with animals and their waste, and
as a result of poor hygiene or unsanitary living or eating conditions. A well-balanced diet and healthy lifestyle are especially
important for reducing the risk of parasitic infection, since a
healthy digestive system will usually destroy parasites and worms.
Use of antibiotics, which kill the beneficial flora of the intestines,
can help set up an environment for parasites. Improperly cooked
meat, especially pork, and eating dirt or walking barefoot are
other common sources of infestation.

Pinworms are the most common parasites in children and are
easily spread when the child scratches around the anus and then
touches another person or object. Symptoms may include bad
breath, dark circles under the eyes, paleness around the mouth,
nose picking, itchy anus, grinding the teeth and waking in the

night. Pinworms can be detected by inspecting the anus with a flashlight several hours after a child has gone to sleep. At this time the female, which looks like a white thread about one-quarter inch long, will crawl out to lay eggs. If there is any doubt about what you're seeing, use a piece of scotch tape to trap a sample. During treatment, avoid all sugar and sweeteners, since worms love them. Acidophilus supplements, or yogurt containing live cultures, can help to restore the balance of intestinal flora, especially following use of antibiotics. Wash and change bedding, pajamas, and underwear daily, and make sure that hands are frequently washed, especially after going to the bathroom or touching the bottom. Underwear should be worn while sleeping.

Roundworm, hookworm, and tapeworm are more serious parasitic infestations that require constitutional and/or medical treatment by a qualified practitioner.

Herbs: Pumpkin seeds; raw garlic, pomegranate, figs, almonds, and **papaya** are vermifuge or antiparasitic foods; fresh **carrot** juice before meals; **black walnut** kills parasites in the digestive system but should not be used by infants or small children; **cascara sagrada,** helps eliminate waste; **cayenne,** with yogurt, for older children who can handle it; **echinacea/goldenseal,** helps destroy parasites and worms; **horsetail,** kills worms and their eggs; **tansy** or **wormwood** tea, for intestinal parasites; also **fennel, mint, sage, slippery elm,** or **thyme** tea.

Homeopathics: Chelone tincture, one to five drops, described in the homeopathic materia medica as "an enemy to every kind of worm infesting the human body," especially indicated for round and pinworms; **Cina,** the classic homeopathic remedy for suspected pinworm infestation, with irritability, nosepicking, dark circles, teeth-grinding, swollen abdomen; **Filix mas,** especially if tapeworm is suspect, with bloating, gnawing pain, worse from eating sweets, digestive upsets including diarrhea, constipation, or vomiting, itchy nose, blue rings around eyes, swollen lymph glands; **Granatum,** for suspicion of tapeworm, with constant hunger, pain around belly button, itchy anus and palms, sunken eyes, vertigo or nausea; **Ratanhia,** for pinworms, with intense pain, heat, or itching of anus; **Santonin,** for night cough, bad breath, itchy nose, dark rings around the eyes, possible colorblindness, teeth-grinding, restless sleep and/or bedwetting;

Spigelia, for bad breath, runny nose, itchy anus, pain around belly button, child may be afraid of pointed objects, such as pins; **Teucrium,** for bad breath, restless sleep, crawling feeling in rectal area after bowel; **Viola odorata,** for worms in children, symptoms may be accompanied by tension and burning in the forehead, dislike of music, milky, strong smelling urine, and possibly bedwetting.

Flower Essences: Crab Apple.

Essential Oils: In bath or massage, as preventive, **bergamot, chamomile, eucalyptus, fennel, lavender, santolina (lavender cotton), lemon, niaouli, peppermint, terebinth,** or **thyme;** in diffuser, any of the above, as well as **caraway, cinnamon,** or **clove;** add **eucalyptus** or **lavender essence** to an ointment applied to the anus before bed, to relieve itching and discourage egg-laying by pinworms.

POISON IVY/OAK/SUMAC

Volatile oils in the bark, roots, leaves, and stems of these plants cause an itchy, inflamed rash within hours or days of exposure. The rash can last for several days or weeks and appears wherever the oil was rubbed. The response is an allergic one that can worsen with each exposure. If these plants are burned, the smoke can also cause inflammations, even in the mouth and nasal passages. Wash immediately with soap and water following suspected exposure, then wipe with alcohol to remove any trace of volatile oil. Powdered green clay can be used as a plaster to soothe itching, as can wheat bran. Cucumber slices can also be laid on the rash. Warm baths with oatmeal or baking soda and hot showers or ice packs may help relieve itching.

Herbs: Plantain or **grindelia juice** can be used as an external wash or poultice, either from freshly crushed leaves or in tincture form; **calendula** tincture or infusion, or **sage** or diluted **lemon** juice can be used externally as a wash; **comfrey root** and **slippery elm** powder can be used as a poultice; **echinacea** and **garlic** can be taken internally to boost immunity and lessen infection; **milkweed** juice can be applied externally; **sage,** as tea or infusion, added to a warm bath can be soothing.

Homeopathics: Anacardium, for poison ivy or poison oak, very itchy, burns after being scratched, especially if eruptions are on the face, better after eating; **Graphites,** for rash that oozes golden fluid, worse at night and from warmth; **Ledum,** immediately after exposure as a preventative, or for rash that feels better after cool applications; **Rhus tox,** for poison ivy, scratching or bathing make rash worse, also more bothersome at night; **Rhus diversiloba,** for poison oak; **Sulfur,** for burning, itching rash made worse by warmth, may scratch until it bleeds.

RESPIRATORY PROBLEMS (Colds, Flu, Bronchitis, Cough, Rhinitis, Sinusitis, Sore Throat)

Because many respiratory conditions tend to have similar symptoms and respond to similar treatments, I will discuss them all here. Respiratory problems are usually caused by viruses or bacteria, although they can also be triggered by irritants in the air or allergies to foods or chemicals. Respiratory conditions affect the mucous membranes of the upper respiratory tract—the nose, nasal passages and cavity, pharynx, and larynx; and the lower respiratory tract—the windpipe, bronchial tubes, lungs, and pleura.

Common colds are characterized by a stuffy, runny nose, known as rhinitis. The infection may spread to the pharynx and cause a sore throat as well, and may be accompanied by a cough. Flus are generally distinguished from the common cold by more serious and uncomfortable symptoms, such as an all-over feeling of achiness and extreme fatigue. Sinusitis is characterized by inflammation and pain in the sinuses and the air spaces in the bones above the eyes and around the nose. Bed rest, eliminating mucus-causing foods such as dairy products, peanuts, sugar, and bananas, drinking plenty of liquids, and vitamin C and zinc supplements are all helpful in speeding recovery from respiratory conditions. If symptoms persist or are accompanied by a high fever, consult your physician.

Herbs: Aniseed, for sore throat, dry cough; **balm of Gilead,** as an expectorant to increase productivity of cough; **echinacea,** immediately on onset of symptoms to boost immune response; **elder flowers, peppermint,** and **yarrow,** individually or in combination; **elecampane,** an expectorant; **garlic,** fresh or in capsules; **goldenseal,** an antimicrobial, for bronchitis and sinusitis;

licorice root, demulcent (soothing) qualities as well as expectorant, antiviral, and antimicrobial actions (do not take for longer than four to six weeks); **lime blossom/linden tree flower/tilia tea** has been found to be more effective than antibiotics in reducing the severity and length of suffering in childhood respiratory diseases; **marshmallow,** anti-inflammatory, to ease sore throat or dry cough, sinusitis; **mullein,** for irritated throat or cough; **sage,** antimicrobial, contains astringents called tannins that help reduce inflammation of a sore throat, infusion makes a good gargle, though the taste may be too strong for children; **thyme,** a powerful antibacterial, antifungal, immune system stimulant, expectorant and respiratory relaxant, can be used as a tea, mouthwash, or gargle for all conditions including bronchitis; **white horehound,** expectorant; **wild cherry bark,** to soothe sore throat or dry cough.

Homeopathics: Aconite, at first sign of cold or sore throat, sudden onset with fever and restlessness, one cheek may be red, the other pale, sneezing, stuffy nose; **Allium cepa,** colds that come on in damp, cold weather, sneezing after entering a warm room, may wake up at 2 A.M., worse in evening and warm, stuffy rooms, better in open air; **Antimonium tartaricum,** for whiny, clingy behavior in child, mucus rattling in chest, but little is coughed up, bronchitis, may be very sleepy and crave acidic fruits and cold water; **Belladonna,** for dry, tickling cough, worse at night, hoarseness, painful larynx, sinusitis with headache that may be worse on right side; **Bryonia,** for sinus headache, with irritability, soreness in larynx and windpipe, hoarseness, dry cough worse at night and after entering a warm room; **Causticum,** for cough with little expectoration that is swallowed, hoarseness, raw pain in chest, voice seems to echo, better from drinking cold water, may be drowsy in daytime and wakeful at night; **Euphrasia,** for watery eyes with discharge, yawning, coughing with much expectoration in the morning, flu, may gag when clearing throat; **Ferrum phos,** at first stage of head colds, especially for nervous or anemic people predisposed to colds, bronchitis in children, may be a gritty feeling in the eyes, sore throat, tonsillitis, symptoms worse at night, 4 A.M. to 6 A.M., **Hepar sulph,** for sneezing and runny nose from going into cold, dry wind, sinusitis, loss of voice, hoarse, dry cough, worse in the morning and when walking, from eating cold food, or whenever an exposed body part feels cold or wind; **Ipecac,** for constriction in chest, wheezing, sneezing, incessant, violent, unproductive cough, croup, worse from warm, moist wind, especially for overweight kids or grownups or those who tend to catch cold while on vacation; **Kali bich,** for hacking cough with sticky yellow expectoration, worse in the evening, tickling in larynx, croup, sniffles in fat babies, violent sneezing, recurrent sinusitis; **Natrum mur,** for sinusitis, runny nose with clear discharge that changes to stuffed up nose after a few days, a cold that starts with sneezing, loss of senses of smell and taste, cough with headache that feels like tickling in the pit of the stomach, worse about 10 A.M.; **Phosphorus,** for sore throat that makes it difficult or impossible to talk, tickling or coughing when talking, worse in cold air and from strong odors or presence of strangers, while reading or laughing, heat in the chest, possibly accompanied by head congestion; **Phytolacca,** for dark or bluish red throat with pain in the soft palate and root of tongue, tonsillitis, especially right tonsil swollen, shooting pain with swallowing, can't tolerate swallowing anything hot, dry, ticklish cough, worse at night; **Pulsatilla,** for hoarseness that comes and goes, dry cough at night, must sit up in bed, expectoration in the morning, soreness and feeling of pressure on chest, feeling of being suffocated on lying down, weepy, enjoying attention and caresses; **Sulfur,** for difficulty breathing, wants to open windows, rattling cough, worse from talking, feeling of heat and weight on chest, greenish, sweet expectoration.

Flower Essences: A child's emotions vary during illness. **Aspen** or **Mimulus** can be useful if there is underlying fearfulness or anxiety. Read the list at the end of Chapter 4 to determine which essences will best help your child's emotional state.

Essential Oils: Ginger, in baths, to increase resistance; **eucalyptus, peppermint, pine, rosemary, tea tree,** in baths, massage, and inhalations; **thyme,** used in a diffuser or steam inhalation, relaxes the bronchials, increases the fluidity of phlegm, and promotes its expulsion; for cough, **eucalyptus, benzoin, fennel, hyssop,** or **sandalwood;** for bronchitis, in inhalation, **eucalyptus, pine,** or **thyme;** for sore throat, in inhalation, **benzoin, lavender, sandalwood,** or **thyme.**
See also: Allergies, Asthma, Stress, Whooping Cough

Ringworm

Ringworm is actually a fungal infection that spreads out in a circle, causing a reddish, circle-shaped eruption. The most important thing to do during treatment is keep very clean. If it fails to heal, consult your practitioner.

Herbs: Tinctures of **calendula, chaparral, echinacea, goldenseal,** or **myrrh** can be applied directly to the site several times a day.

Homeopathics: Graphites, for ringworm with sticky, golden crusts, possibly also bad-smelling foot perspiration; **Rhus tox,** for humid ringworm, especially on scalp or face; **Sepia,** for itchy or brown ringworm, may be worse at knees and elbows, possibly recurring in springtime; **Sulfur,** for dry, red, irritated, itchy, worse from scratching.

Flower Essences: Crab Apple.

Essential Oils: In the bath, **lavender, myrrh,** or **tea tree;** any of these three applied directly to the infection.

Skin Problems (Eczema, Psoriasis, Rashes, Warts)

Many natural practitioners equate the health of the skin with the state of overall health. Skin problems have many causes, from nervous or emotional stress to immune system problems from toxins in the environment. Poor diet and allergies can also be factors. Whenever skin problems appear, look first to the diet, cutting out common problem foods such as fatty or processed foods, meat, sugar, and fruit juices. Soothing baths that include oatmeal, barley water, or baking soda can be helpful as well.

Herbs: To get rid of warts, peel a **garlic** clove, slice in half, and place the cut side of the garlic directly against the wart, holding it there with gauze or tape. Replace with a fresh piece of garlic two or three times a day until the wart burns off. **Dandelion** juice or a **banana** skin poultice may also help get rid of warts. **Burdock, nettle, sarsaparilla, dandelion, dock,** or **echinacea,** in tea infusion or tincture, can be helpful to the body during skin ailments; **calendula** cream or ointment to soothe and heal; **urtica** lotion or ointment to soothe itching; **chamomile** infusion for bathing.

Homeopathics: Anacardium, for intensely itchy eczema with irritability, for warts on hands, also for poison oak; **Arsenicum album,** for dry, rough, scaly skin, worse from scratching and from cold, psoriasis, may be worse on the right side and after midnight; **Bovista,** for rashes from nervous excitement, itching, moist, crusty eczema, especially on back of hand, perspiration may have smell of onions; **Calcarea carb,** for rashes and small wounds that don't heal, warts on face and hands, symptoms may be worse at full moon, especially for fat, fair, flabby kids who are very sensitive to cold; **Calendula,** for eczema, especially in infants; **Croton tiglium,** for intense itching that hurts to scratch, herpes zoster, worse during summer, night and morning, and from touch or washing; **Oleander,** for extremely sensitive skin that chaps or irritates easily, violent itching, sensitive scalp, herpes, pimples; **Ruta graveolens,** for aftereffects of frostbite; **Silicea,** helps to dislodge splinters; **Sulfur,** for dry, unhealthy, itchy skin, worse from scratching or washing; **Vinca minor,** for itchy, moist eczema of the scalp and face, skin sensitive, reddens from slightest rubbing, hair may be matted, also for common warts: **Antimonium crudum, Causticum, Nitric acidum,** or **Thuja,** for warts; **Mercurius,** for plantar warts.

Flower Essences: Crab Apple, for cleansing; **Five Flower** or **Rescue Remedy** cream or tincture; other flower essences as appropriate to the individual. See end of Chapter 4.

Essential Oils: For eczema, **chamomile, hyssop, melissa,** or **sage;** for dry eczema, **geranium** or **lavender;** for weeping eczema, **juniper;** for dermatitis, **chamomile, geranium, hyssop, juniper, sage,** or **thyme;** for psoriasis, **bergamot, lavender,** or **sandalwood;** for pimples, **lavender** can be applied undiluted; **onion** essential oil, for chapped or cracked skin; **lemon,** for oily skin; a drop of **lemon** or **tea tree** can be applied directly to a wart, several times a day until it disappears.
See also: STRESS

STRESS

Although a certain amount of stress in life is inevitable and may even provide motivation for change, excessive stress can tear down basic health and immune response, and, over time, can lead to stress-related disorders such as allergies, asthma, depression, digestive complaints, eczema and psoriasis, headaches, insomnia, and heart disease. Meditation, prayer, creative hobbies, deep breathing, and exercise can have a beneficial effect on our ability to cope with stress, lending greater emotional balance, peace of mind, stamina, and endurance. Vitamins B and C can be rapidly depleted under stressful conditions, and should be supplemented as necessary.

Herbs: Nervine herbs, such as **borage, chamomile, lavender, lemon balm, lime flowers, oats, orange blossom, passion-flower, rose petals, skullcap,** and **verbena,** can be taken as tea for strengthening and toning the nervous system; **ginseng,** an adaptogen, helps the body to deal with the effects of stress.

Homeopathics: Arnica, after intense mental strain or shock; **Arsenicum,** for burnout, with feelings of anguish, restlessness, and despair, when even the slightest exertion causes feelings of exhaustion, possibly with great thirst but aversion to food; **Carbolicum acidum,** for difficulty concentrating on mental tasks, craving for tobacco and stimulants, also may be bad breath, heightened sense of smell, and headaches that feel better after smoking; **Ignatia,** for emotional stress resulting from repressed fear, anger, grief, or embarrassment, usually with sighing, insomnia, crying when alone, worse from sympathy and tobacco smoke, better after eating; **Natrum mur,** for illness following emotional stress, rejection, castigation, or disappointment, startled and upset by sudden noises, worse at 10 A.M. and in the sun, better in the open air; **Nux vomica,** for stress resulting from mental strain and sedentary lifestyle, with irritability and fault-finding behavior; **Ruta graveolens,** for stress, fatigue, and eyestrain, possibly with carpal tunnel symptoms, from too much time spent in front of a computer screen.

Flower Essences: Agrimony, for stress hidden behind a cheerful facade; **Centaury,** for stress as a result of overdoing for others, the "doormat" remedy; **Cherry Plum,** when stress overstrains the mind, giving rise to desperate thoughts and tendencies; **Elm,** for those who are following their calling in life but are temporarily overwhelmed and feel they have taken on too much; **Hornbeam,** for the feeling of not having enough strength in body or mind to deal with what needs to be done; **Oak,** for "fighters" who are under a great deal of stress but keep going, sometimes to the breaking point; **Olive,** for exhaustion following periods of intense stress and struggle; **Rock Rose,** for the stress of sudden trauma or bad news; **Star of Bethlehem,** for spiritual comfort following shock or loss; **Sweet Chestnut,** for anguish, the "dark night of the soul"; **White Chestnut,** when stress results in unceasing circular thinking or uncontrollable repetitive thoughts that distract one from focusing on the present and destroy peace of mind; **Five Flower** or **Rescue Remedy.**

Essential Oils: Calming, uplifting essences include **basil, bergamot, chamomile, clary sage, geranium, jasmine, lavender, marjoram, neroli, rose, sandalwood,** and **ylang-ylang,** in massage and in the bath. **Cypress, rosemary,** and **sage** help to balance the nervous system. **Ginger, lemongrass,** and **rosemary** help strengthen the adrenals, which become exhausted and weakened under prolonged stress.

Sunburn: see Burns

Teething

A baby's first teeth usually appear around the age of four to six months and are often accompanied by crankiness, pulling or rubbing on the ears, drooling, a cheek that is red on the side of the erupting tooth, chewing on everything within reach, runny nose, waking up at night or having trouble getting to sleep, and crying for no apparent reason. Cold objects or a clean, cool, wet cloth can be given to the baby to chew on to relieve the discomfort of the new tooth pushing through the gum.

Herbs: Catnip, chamomile, or **lemon balm** tea can help to calm and relax, and a cloth can be soaked in the cold tea for the baby to suck on; **lobelia** can be rubbed onto the gums; **marshmallow** root syrup can be given, one teaspoon three times daily; **meadowsweet** tincture for relief of inflamed gums.

Homeopathics: Chamomilla is probably the most commonly used homeopathic remedy; **Belladonna,** for a high fever, tendency to bite, teeth and gums red, or when Chamomilla doesn't work; **Calcarea carb,** for late onset of teething, baby puts fingers in mouth to relieve pain, baby is pudgy, head may perspire, bodily fluids smell sour; **Calcarea phos,** for late onset of teething in thin or slow-growing infant; **Coffea,** when baby is too restless to sleep or awakens in the middle of the night with teething pain; **Cypripedium,** when the child wakes at night to laugh and play; **Kreosote,** for irritability and summer diarrhea, worse from cold food, better from a hot meal; **Phytolacca,** when child presses teeth or gums together, tip of tongue may be red.

Flower Essences: Five Flower or **Rescue Remedy** may be rubbed into the gums.

Essential Oils: A drop of **blue chamomile** in a teaspoon of carrier oil may be massaged into the affected side of the face; a drop of **lavender, mandarin, marjoram,** or **neroli** in a bowl of hot water next to baby's bed promotes calm sleep.

URINARY TRACT INFECTION

Because the urethra is very short in women, they have a much greater tendency to infections of the urinary tract than do men. Symptoms include frequent urges to urinate, though little urine is excreted, burning pain with urination, cloudy or bloody urine, and pain, cramping, or tenderness in the lower abdomen or back. Avoiding caffeine, perfumed feminine hygiene products, polyester underwear, and artificial perfumes or dyes in soaps and bubble baths can help prevent infections from occurring, as can urinating after sexual intercourse. Once you've noticed symptoms, drink lots of liquids to flush out bacteria. Cranberry juice is an effective and well-known home remedy, although it is not the acidity that accounts for its effectiveness but an unexplained property of the juice that makes it difficult for the bacteria to adhere to the walls of the bladder and multiply. Infections can cause complications by spreading to the kidneys or bloodstream and should not be neglected. If symptoms are not gone within two days, or if symptoms include high fever, weakness, or back pain, consult your physician.

Herbs: Bearberry, the active ingredient in which is arbutin, which is converted to hydroquinone, has antiseptic effects on the urinary passages. (Do not use vitamin C or cranberry juice while taking this herb, as it cancels out the effect.) Instead try **corn silk** as a diuretic and demulcent herb that can help ease the uncomfortable symptoms of the infection without interfering with the action of the bearberry); **chamomile** tea is another good liquid to drink, and **garlic,** fresh or in capsules, helps to fight infection.

Homeopathics: Aconite, at very first awareness of symptoms; **Apis,** for burning pain, worse at night and from heat, abdomen is very sensitive, better from cold; **Berberis,** for cutting pains during or after urinating, worse from movement; **Cantharis,** for frequent urges with scanty output and burning during urination; **Mercurius,** for burning pain, worst just before or after urinating rather than during; **Nux vomica,** when symptoms may come on after overindulgence in food, coffee, alcoholic beverages, or drugs, with burning or pressing pain in the bladder and/or urethra; **Pulsatilla,** for infections in those who have the classic Pulsatilla personality type (sweet, calm, quiet, enjoy hugs and sympathy), symptoms worse lying on the back, may be dribbling of urine while coughing, sneezing, laughing, or being startled; **Sarsaparilla,** when pain is greatest at the end of urinating.

Essential Oils: Bergamot, chamomile, eucalyptus, juniper, sandalwood, or **tea tree,** in hot compresses to the lower abdomen.

WARTS: see Skin Problems

WHOOPING COUGH (PERTUSSIS)

The early symptoms of whooping cough are similar to those of a common cold, but after about a week, a violent cough, sometimes to the point of vomiting, sets in, usually at night. This highly contagious infection usually occurs in children, and the "whoop" is the sound they make while trying to catch their breath. There is a vaccine for pertussis, but there is some controversy regarding its effectiveness and potential side effects. Whooping cough in babies and children under the age of two years can sometimes cause choking and oxygen deprivation, or progress into pneumonia, which can damage the lungs, so be sure to consult with your pediatrician. A child with whooping cough should be kept away from other children for at least a month and should not be allowed anywhere near babies or toddlers. Those suffering from this condition should not be left alone, as there is a danger of suffocation from inhaling expectorated or vomited material.

Herbs: To fight infection and strengthen the lungs, an infusion of **aniseed, coltsfoot, ginger, horehound, hyssop, licorice, sage,** or **thyme; lemon balm** tea for calming; **garlic,** crushed and wrapped in cotton and applied as a poultice to the feet to aid expectoration, remove after fifteen minutes.

Homeopathics: Aconite or **Belladonna,** in first stage for cough; **Bryonia,** for dry, painful cough, child has difficulty eating; **Coccus cacti,** for coughs that produce tough, white mucus that may stick in the throat and cause feelings of strangulation, brushing teeth brings on coughing, tickling in larynx, constant swallowing, uvula swollen, may be worse upon waking up; **Drosera,** Hahnemann's principal remedy for whooping cough, for deep, hoarse coughing fits with choking and difficulty breathing, to the point of retching, yellow expectoration, possibly blood-streaked, worse after midnight, coughing may start at bedtime; **Euphrasia,** daytime only, with much watering from the eyes; **Ipecacuanha,** for violent coughing, trouble catching breath, becomes stiff and blue in the face, may be accompanied by nosebleed, getting worse periodically and from lying down; **Natrum mur,** for coughing accompanied by flow of tears.

Flower Essences: Five Flower or **Rescue Remedy** to restore calm.

Essential Oils: In inhalation or vaporizer, **cypress, lavender, rosemary, tea tree,** or **thyme; thyme,** well-diluted in the bath; use any of the preceding oils in massage of chest and back.

YEAST AND THRUSH

Candida albicans, a fungus that can manifest as thrush in the mouth or as a vaginal yeast infection, commonly appears as a side effect of the use of antibiotics, which are effective against bacteria but do not kill fungi. Babies or children may get small white patches inside the mouth or on the tongue that later turn raw and red and may bleed. Vaginal yeast can be sexually transmitted, or occur during pregnancy or while taking birth control pills. Poor nutrition or fatigue can also open the system to attack by this organism. Yeast thrives on sugar, which should be eliminated from the diet. Yogurt which contains live acidophilus cultures can be eaten or applied inside the vaginal canal. Douching with a solution of vinegar can also bring results by restoring the acidic balance.

Herbs: Infusion or tincture of **calendula, echinacea,** or **ladies' mantle,** internally; **calendula, goldenseal,** or **lavender infusion** externally as a wash or mouthwash.

Homeopathics: Borax, especially in nursing baby, mouth is dry and hurts; **Kali mur,** for coated tongue, white ulcers in mouth, glands may be swollen, thick, nonirritating milky white vaginal discharge; **Mercurius,** bad breath, sore mouth, puffy tongue, bleeding gums; **Natrum mur,** pearl-like sores in mouth, watery, burning vaginal discharge; **Pulsatilla,** for creamy, burning vaginal discharge; **Sulfur,** for sore, red, burning mouth, if **Mercurius** doesn't work.

Flower Essences: Metaphysically, yeast infections are correlated with difficulty in standing up for one's own needs. **Centaury** and **Cerato** can be of some assistance in supporting the sense of self.

Essential Oils: Geranium, lavender, lemon, myrrh, sage, or **tea tree** in baths.

NATIVE AMERICAN COMMANDMENTS

∽ Treat the earth and all that dwell thereon with respect.

∽ Remain close to the Great Spirit.

∽ Show great respect to your fellow beings.

∽ Work together for the benefit of all Mankind.

∽ Give assistance and kindness wherever needed.

∽ Do what you know to be right.

∽ Look after the well-being of mind and body.

∽ Dedicate a share of your efforts to the greater good.

∽ Be truthful and honest at all times.

∽ Take full responsibility for your actions.

Resource Guide

Freeze-Frame Technique

Institute of Heartmath, A Nonprofit Corporation
Doc Lew Childre
P.O. Box 1463/14700 West Park Ave.
Boulder Creek, CA 95006
(408) 338-8700
e-mail: hrtmath@netcom.com
Seminars and classes, also books and tapes, including *Teaching Children to Love* and *Freeze Frame.*

Scientific research and numerous case studies show Freeze-Frame is effective in releasing stress, sadness, and anger and provides a positive, balanced perspective that stimulates creativity and insight. The technique is taught through seminars, books, and tapes available through the Institute of Heartmath, listed above. The basic Freeze-Frame steps are as follows:

- Recognize a stressful feeling/experience and take a "time out"—Freeze-Frame the feeling.

- Shift the attention from the racing mind or disturbed emotions to the area around the heart.

- Activate a warm, pleasant, fun feeling (love for a family member, fun time with friends, and so forth).

- Ask the heart intelligence for a more efficient response to the original situation.

- Listen to what your heart says.

—From Doc Lew Childre's *Teaching Children to Love: 80 Games and Fun Activities for Raising Balanced Children in Unbalanced Times,* Boulder Creek, Calif.: Planetary Publications. Used with permission.

Candlemaking

General Wax and Candle
6863 Beck Ave.
North Hollywood, CA 91605
(818) 765-6357
Beeswax and candle-making supplies.

HERBS

The following are reputable suppliers of seeds, products, books, and classes. Call or write for more information, or for a store or outlet carrying recommended products in your area.

Western United States

Horizon Seeds
Richo and Mayche Cech
P.O. Box 69
Williams, OR 97544-0069
(503) 846-6704
Seeds, many of them ethically wildcrafted, for medicinal herbs.

Eclectic Institute
30900 SE Division Dr.
Troutdale, OR 97060
(503) 668-4120
Herbal extracts, supplements, books, and papers.

The Herb Pharm
Ed Smith
Williams, OR
(503) 846-6262
High-quality tinctures.

The Herbalist
Tierne Salter
2106 N.E. 65th
Seattle, WA 98115
(206) 523-2600
Seattle's main herb store, with tinctures, formulas, and bodycare items.

Jeanne Rose
219 Carl St.
San Francisco, CA 94117
(415) 564-6337
The American First Lady of Herbs, herbal products, formulas, and classes.

Louis J. Marx, M.D.
3418 Loma Vista Rd. #1-A
Ventura, CA 93003
(805) 642-2115
Herbal treatments and neurokinesiology. *Monastery of Herbs* formulas.

Dr. Richard Schulze's School of Natural Healing
P. O. Box 3628
Santa Monica, CA 90408-3628
(310) 576-6565
Classes, correspondence course, herbal products, and formulas.

Herb Products Co.
John Devol
11012 Magnolia Blvd.
North Hollywood, CA 91601
(818) 984-3141
Wide range of dried herbs, and related books and products.

Roses of Yesterday and Today
802 Browns Valley Road
Watsonville, CA 95076
(408) 724-3537
Excellent source for many old rose varieties. Catalog $3.00.

Lavender Lane
7337 #1 Roseville Road
Sacramento, CA 95842
(916) 334-4400
Herbs and herbalware, bottles, labels, beeswax, books, and much more.
Catalog $2.00.

Desert Woman Botanicals
Monica Rude
P.O. Box 263
Gila, NM 88038
(505) 535-2860 (messages)
Grower of herbs, also sells plants.

Southwest Medicinal Plants
Mimi Kamp and Halsey Brant
Box 5
Naco, AZ 85620
(520) 432-2688
Tinctures and flower essences.

Winter Sun Trading Co.
Phyllis Hogan
107 N. San Francisco, Suite #1
Flagstaff, AZ 86001
(602) 774-2884
Wildcrafted and organic tinctures. Southwestern Native American plant specialist.

Southwest School of Botanical Medicine
Michael Moore, director
Donna Chesner, administrator
P.O. Box 4565
Bisbee, AZ 85603
(520) 432-5855

Turtle Island Herbs
Feather Jones
Salina Star Route
Boulder, CO 80302
(303) 442-2215
Tinctures and formulas.

Dancing Willow Herbs
Debra Rueben
960 Main Street
Durango, CO 81302
(970) 247-1654
Retail store, wildcrafted tinctures and tea blends, formulas.

Midwestern United States

Nature's Cathedral
Leroy Ballard
RRT 1 Box 120
Blairstown, IA 52209
(319) 454-6959
Cultivate (rather than wildcraft) echinacea and goldenseal, among other herbs.

Ginseng Business Center
16H Menard Plaza
Wausau, WI 54401
(715) 845-7300
Wisconsin-grown ginseng.

Eastern United States

The University of Natural Healing
355 West Rio Road, Suite 201
Charlottesville, VA 22902
(804) 973-0262
Books and classes.

Southern Virginia Herbals
Robert Wooding
Rt 3 Box 81
Hallfax, VA 24558
(804) 476-1339
Organic and wildcrafted East Coast herbs.

Blessed Herbs
Martha and Michael Volchok
109 Barre Plains Road
Oakham, MA 01068
(800) 489-4372
Wide variety of herbs, including ethically wildcrafted.

David Winston, Herbalist and Alchemist
P.O. Box 553
Broadway, NJ 08808
(908) 689-9020
East Coast herbal tinctures and bulk products.

Susun Weed
P.O. Box 64
Woodstock, NY 12498
(914) 246-8081
Classes, books, apprenticeships.

HOMEOPATHY: Homeopathic Remedies and Education

Homeopathy Overnight
RR1 Box 818
Kingfield, ME 04947
(800) ARNICA 30
Remedies, tinctures, ointments, kits, and books. I have not tried this source, but they advertise that they can send any of five hundred remedies for $9.75, including shipping. Free catalog.

Boericke and Tafel
2381 Circadian Way
Santa Rosa, CA 95407
(707) 571-8202
Remedies, kits, books, and tapes. Products are available in health food stores and natural pharmacies.

Boiron-Bornemann, Inc.
98c West Cochran
Simi Valley, CA 93065
(805) 582-9091
Remedies and kits. Products are available in health food stores and natural pharmacies.

Dolisos
3014 Rigel
Las Vegas, NV 89102
(800) DOLISOS (365-4767)
More than 2,500 classical single remedies. Free catalog.

Historical Remedies
122 S. Wabasha St. Suite 320
St. Paul, MN 55107
(612) 224-9344
Remedies and kits. Free catalog.

Standard Homeopathic Company
154 West 131st St.
Los Angeles, CA 90061
(213) 321-4284
Remedies and books.

National Center for Homeopathy
801 N. Fairfax #306
Alexandria, VA 22314
(703) 548-7790
Coordinates nationwide groups that meet weekly or monthly to share information on homeopathy. Write for information on purchasing a directory of groups or to find a listing in your area.

Homeopathic Education Services
2124 Kittredge St.
Berkeley, CA 94704
(510) 649-0294
Listings of schools and training programs headed by Dana Ullmann.

FLOWER ESSENCES: Flower Essences and Education

Flower Essence Pharmacy
Gary Mason
6600 N. Hwy 1
Little River, CA 95456
(800) 343-8693 (orders)
(707) 937-5059 (information)
web page: www.floweressences.com
The single most comprehensive source for flower essences that I know of, with a selection of more than 4,000 essences from 50 different companies located in more than 15 different countries, as well as a wide variety of books. Their 1,000-page catalog can be downloaded as a compressed file if you are online.

Flower Essence Society
Patricia Kaminski
P.O. Box 1769
Nevada City, CA 95959
(800) 548 0075
e-mail: orders@floweressence.com
web page: www.floweressence.com
Sierra wildflower essences, Healing Herbs (Bach flower essences made by Julian and Martine Barnard), books and classes.

Star Essence
Star Riparetti
312 W. Yanonali St.
Santa Barbara, CA 93101
(805) 965-1619
Flower essences made from Peruvian orchids and Santa Barbara wildflowers, books, and classes.

Alaskan Flower Essence Project
P.O. Box 1369
Homer, AK 99603
(907) 235-2188
Flower essences and gem elixirs from Alaska. Free catalog.

Perelandra
Machaelle Small Wright
P.O. Box 3603
Warrenton, VA 22186
Flower essences, books, and classes.

AROMATHERAPY: Essential Oils, Aromatherapy Products, Education, and Publications

Western United States

Aromatherapy Quarterly
#238, P.O. Box 421
Inverness, CA 94937-0421
(415) 663-9128
English aromatherapy journal founded by aromatherapist Patricia Davis.

The International Journal of Aromatherapy
P.O. Box 750428
Petaluma, CA 94975-0428
(800) 809-9850
Excellent quarterly magazine founded by Robert Tisserand.

Aromatherapy Seminars/Laboratory of Flowers
Michael Scholes and Joan Clark
117 N. Robertson Blvd.
Los Angeles, CA 90048
(800) 677-2368
Essential oils, perfume absolutes, products, books, classes, correspondence course.

Aroma Vera
Los Angeles, CA
5901 Rodeo Rd.
Los Angeles, CA 90016-4312
(800) 669-9514
Essential oils, aromatherapy products, available in many health food stores and salons. Complimentary guide and introductory special.

Elizabeth Van Buren Aromatherapy
303 Potrero St. #33
Santa Cruz, CA 95060
(800) 710-7759
Spectrix GC/MS Lab tested essential oils, aromatherapy products.

Original Swiss Aromatics/Pacific Institute of Aromatherapy
Kurt Schnaubelt
P.O. Box 6723
San Rafael, CA 94903
(415) 479-9121
Essential oils, aromatherapy products, education, and conferences.

Oshadi
15 Monarch Bay Plaza Suite 346
Monarch Beach, CA 92629
(800) 933-1008
Quality essential oils and diffusers.

Tisserand Aromatherapy
P.O. Box 750428
Petaluma, CA 94975-0428
(707) 769-5120
Essential oils, aromatherapy products, and books.

Quan Yin Essentials
(707) 431-0529
High quality aromatherapy products.

wives tales
11116 Riverside Dr.
North Hollywood, CA 91602
(800) 955-8253
Aromatherapy for kids, bubble baths, massage oils, and books. Free catalog.

NAHA
P.O. Box 17622
Boulder, CO 80308-7622
(800) 566-6735
National Association for Holistic Aromatherapists, membership organization.

Aromaland Inc.
1326 Rutina Circle
Santa Fe, NM 84505
(800) 933-5267
Essential oils, diffusers, and aromatherapy products. Free catalog.

Midwestern United States

The Aromatic Thymes
75 Lakeview Parkway
Barrington, IL 60010
(847) 526-0456
Pam Parsons, editor
$30/yr. subscription to excellent quarterly magazine.

Aromatherapy Services
Pat Nelson
3215 W. Lawrence St.
Appleton, WI 54914
(414) 731-0667
Essential oils, aromatherapy products, classes, and books.

Amrita Aromatherapy
P.O. Box 2178
Fairfield, IA 52556
(515) 410-9651
Essential oils, aromatherapy products.

Sensory Essence
Jan Salko
P.O. Box 87
Island Lake, IL 60042
(847) 526-3645
High-quality essential oils and Bulgarian rose products.

Eastern United States

Quality of Life Associates
Carol Corio
15 Fox Meadow Lane
Dedham, MA 02026
(800) 688-8343
Essential oils, aromatherapy products, books, and classes.

A Woman of Uncommon Scents
Rachel Shapiro
P.O. Box 103
Roxbury, PA 17251
(717) 530-0609
High-quality essential oils.

Earth Harmony
290 Hilderbrand Dr.
Suite B–13
Atlanta, GA 30328
(800) 341-2604 (order line)
Full line of quality essential oils, diffusors.

WEB PAGES

In addition to the above, the following web pages are excellent sources
of on-line information on natural healing:

www.fragrant.demon.co.uk
Graham Sorenson's Guide to Aromatherapy
Descriptions of essential oils and their listings, books, and more.

www.ars-grin.gov/~ngr/sbl
Agricultural Research Service
Phytochemical and Ethnobotanical Databases
Descriptions of plants used for food and medicinal purposes,
their chemical constituents, and traditional applications.

www.med.uni-muenchen.de/fachschaft/homeopathy/science.htm
Abstracts of studies conducted with homeopathic remedies for a
wide variety of purposes.

http://indy4.fdl.cc.mn.us/~isk/mainmenu.html#mainmenutop
Native American Resources Main Menu
A huge offering of more than 300 web pages, including contemporary
and historical narratives, stories, recipes, and all things cultural for native
peoples of North and South America.

http://chili.rt66.com/hrbmoore/HOMEPAGE/HomePage.html
Southwest School of Botanical Medicine Home Page
Created by Michael Moore, director of the school in Bisbee, Arizona, this site
has *lots* of information on medicinal plants and their uses.

NOTES

CHAPTER ONE Earth Awareness and Natural Health: An Overview

1. Public Interest Research Groups, Internet Paper, August 8, 1997.
2. K.B. Thomas and T. Colborn, "Organochlorine endocrine disrupters in human tissue, Chemically induced alteration in sexual and functional development: The Wildlife/Human connection," (Princeton, New Jersey: Princeton Scientific Publication Co., 1992).
3. T. Colborn, D. Dumanoski, and J. P. Myers, *Our Stolen Future: Are We Threatening Our Fertility, Intelligence, and Survival?* (New York: Dutton, 1996).
4. Stephen B. Edelson M.D., "Can a Poisoned Environment Play a Major Role in the Ability of a Child to Learn?" Internet Paper, 1995.
5. J. L. Jacobsen et al., "Effects of in-utero exposure to polychlorinated biphenyls and related contaminants on cognitive functioning in young children," *Journal of Pediatrics* 116:38–45, 1990.
6. Ann Misch, "Chemical Reaction," *World Watch,* March/April p. 10, 1993.
7. Samer Muscali, "Arctic Home of the Inuit Threatened by Pollution," *Perspectives,* Internet Paper, 1997.
8. Walter J. Rogan M.D. in *Archives of Pediatrics and Adolescent Medicine* 150:981–990, September 1996.
9. Michael Greger, "Bovine Growth Hormone—What You May Not Know," *AnimaLife,* vol. 5, no. 2, Cornell University, Spring, 1995.
10. Nick Nuttall, "Baby Milk Formulas Contain Phthalate," *Times* (London), May 28, 1996.
11. Press Release, Environmental Working Group, "New Alliance Forms to Curb Pesticide Contamination of Midwestern Tap Water," August 12, 1997.
12. Ibid.
13. Children's Environmental Health Network, "What Is Pediatric Environmental Health?" June 1996.
14. Virginia Tech Green Engineering Project, September 16, 1996.
15. Pesticide Action Network North America, August 29, 1997.
16. Ibid.
17. *Sacramento Bee,* September 22, 1997.
18. James C. Robinson et al., California Policy Seminar, "Pesticides in the Home and Community: Health Risks," vol. 6, no. 2, Berkeley, California, April, 1994.
19. Ibid.
20. Ibid.
21. Public Interest Research Groups, "Toxic Right to Know Campaign" paper, August 8, 1997.
22. Rachel Carson, *Silent Spring,* (Boston: Houghton Mifflin Co., 1962).
23. Linda Callahan, "The Crisis of Infertility and Its Effect on the Couple Relationship," *Progress: Family Systems Research and Therapy,* Encino, Calif., vol. 3, pp. 19–35, 1994.
24. Centers for Disease Control, National Center for Health Statistics, "Healthy People 2000," 1996.
25. Virginia Tech Engineering Project, Internet Paper, September 16, 1996.
26. Centers for Disease Control, National Center for Health Statistics, "Healthy People 2000," 1996.
27. Natural Resources Defense Council Report, "Breath-taking: Premature Mortality Due to Particulate Air Pollution in 239 American Cities," May 1996.
28. Natural Resources Defense Council Report, "Out of Breath: Children's Health and Air Pollution in Southern California," 1993.
29. Sabin Russell, "Puzzling Rise in Asthma Deaths," *San Francisco Chronicle,* July 3, 1996.
30. Children's Environmental Health Network, "What Is Pediatric Environmental Health?" June 1996.
31. Sabin Russell, "Puzzling Rise in Asthma Deaths," *San Francisco Chronicle,* July 3, 1996.

32. Ibid.

33. Edelson, Stephen B., M.D. "Can a Poisoned Environment Play a Major Role in the Ability of a Child to Learn?" Internet Paper, 1995.

34. Rain Forest Action Network, "Deforestation Rates in Tropical Forests and Their Climatic Implications," 1997.

35. Norman Myers, "Trees by the Billions: A Blueprint for Ecology," *International Wildlife,* 25:12–15, 1991.

36. Rain Forest Action Network, "Deforestation Rates in Tropical Forests and Their Climatic Implications," 1997.

37. Ibid.

38. D. Satcher Ph.D., "Emerging Infectious Disease Threats," Centers for Disease Control and Prevention Brochure, 1996.

39. Ibid.

40. Ibid.

41. Craig Turner, "Antibiotic-Resistant TB a New Peril, U.N. Says," *Los Angeles Times,* October 23, 1997.

42. Laurie Garrett, *The Coming Plague: Newly Emerging Diseases in a World Out of Balance,* (New York: Penguin, 1996).

43. NCHS Press Release, "HHS Issues Annual Health, United States Report, with Special Profile of Women's Health," June 18, 1996.

44. D. Satcher, "Emerging Infectious Disease Threats," Centers for Disease Control and Prevention Brochure, 1996.

45. Ibid.

46. Consortium for International Science Information Network, "Suppression of the Immune System from Increased Ultraviolet-B Exposure Due to Ozone Depletion," October 29, 1997.

47. Ibid.

48. Francisco Robles, "Casos de colera en Acapulco," *La Opinion,* October 14, 1997.

49. Dawn Kent, U.S. Department of Agriculture BSE Fact Sheet, March 1997.

50. Ibid.

51. Michael Greger, "More Serious Than AIDS," *Earth Island Journal,* vol. 11, no. 3, Summer 1996.

52. WHO Press Release, April 3, 1996.

53. Michael Greger, "The Public Health Implications of Mad Cow Disease," *AnimaLife,* vol. 6, no. 2, Cornell University, Spring 1996.

54. Dawn Kent, U.S. Department of Agriculture BSE Fact Sheet, March 1997.

55. Collinge et al., "The Smoking Gun of BSE," *Nature,* vol. 350, no. 6650, October 2, 1997.

56. James Wood, Epidemiology Unit, Animal Health Trust, Newmarket UK, Internet Paper, 1997.

57. British Department of Health, Monthly CJD Statistical Figures, through September 1997.

58. CDC Report, Meeting on CJD and BSE, April 8, 1996.

59. J. Stauber and S. Rampton, "The U.S. Mad Cow Cover-up," *Earth Island Journal,* vol. 11, no. 3, Summer 1996.

60. Michael Greger, "The Public Health Implications of Mad Cow Disease," *AnimaLife,* vol. 6, no. 2, Cornell University, Spring 1996.

61. J. Stauber and S. Rampton, "The U.S. Mad Cow Cover-up," *Earth Island Journal,* vol. 11, no. 3, Summer 1996.

62. Ibid.

63. Michael Greger, "More Serious Than AIDS," *Earth Island Journal,* vol. 11, no. 3, Summer 1996.

64. D. Satcher, "Emerging Infectious Disease Threats," Centers for Disease Control and Prevention Brochure, 1996.

65. Vladimir Poponin, "The DNA Phantom Effect: Direct Measurement of a New Field in the Vacuum Substructure." Institute of Heart Math Research Papers, May 15, 1995.

66. Lynn Grodski, LCSW, "The Emotional Body: An Interview with Candace Pert, Ph.D.," 1996. Quoted with permission.

67. Referred to in *Doctor's Guide to Medical News,* April 7, 1996.

68. Rollin McCraty et al., "The Effects of Emotions on Short-term Power Spectrum Analysis of Heart Rate Variability," *American Journal of Cardiology,* vol. 76, no. 14, pp. 1089–1093, November 15, 1995.

69. E. M. Widdowson, "Mental Contentment and Physical Growth," *The Lancet,* vol. 1, pp. 1316–1318, 1951; and G. F. Powell et al., "Emotional Deprivation and Growth Retardation Simulating Ediopathic Hypopituitarism," *New England Journal of Medicine,* 176; pp. 1279–1283, 1967.

70. Bernie S. Siegel, M.D., *Love, Medicine, and Miracles: Lessons Learned about Self-Healing from a Surgeon's Experience with Exceptional Patients,* (New York: Harper and Row, 1986).

71. D. Spiegel et al., "Effect of Psychosocial Treatment on Survival of Patients with Metastatic Breast Cancer," *Lancet,* 2, no. 8668, pp. 888–889, October 1989.

72. Bernie S. Siegel, M.D., *Love, Medicine, and Miracles: Lessons Learned about Self-Healing from a Surgeon's Experience with Exceptional Patients,* (New York: Harper and Row, 1986).

73. D. C. McClelland and C. Kirshnit, "The Effects of Motivational Arousal Through Films on Salivary Immunoglobulin A," *Psychological Health,* 2:31–52, 1988.

74. Glen Rein et al., "The Physiological and Psychological Effects of Compassion and Anger," *Journal of Advancement in Medicine,* 8 (2): 87–105, 1995.

75. J. S. House et al., "Social Relationships and Health," *Science,* vol. 241, no. 4865, pp. 540–545, July 1988.

76. L. F. Berkman and S. L. Syme, "Social Networks, Host Resistance, and Mortality: A Nine-Year Follow-Up Study of Alameda County Residents," *American Journal of Epidemiology,* vol. 109, no. 2, pp. 186–204, February 1979.

77. Medical Tribune News Service, "Stress Levels Soar in Working Mothers," *New York Times,* July 24, 1997.

78. Julie A. Hatterer, M.D., "Depression in Women: The Silent Epidemic," *The National Council on Women's Health Newsletter,* Fall 1996.

79. Press Release, Institute of Heart Math, "Are We Reading the Warning Signs? Recent Social Health Statistics Indicate Children Are at Risk," 1996.

80. Randolph C. Byrd, "Positive Therapeutic Effects of Intercessory Prayer in a Coronary Care Unit Population," *Southern Medical Journal,* vol. 81, no. 7, pp. 826–829, July 1988.

81. David B. Larson et al., "The Impact of Religion on Men's Blood Pressure," *Journal of Religion and Health,* vol. 28, pp. 265–278, 1989.

82. "Religious Belief, Depression, and Ambulation Status in Elderly Women with Broken Hips," *American Journal of Psychiatry,* 147:758–760, 1990.

83. Described in: HomeArts Network, "Prayer: The Proof," *Country Living's Healthy Living,* Hearst, 1997.

84. Ibid.

85. W. Braud and M. Schlitz, "Psychokinetic Influence on Electrodermal Activity," *Journal of Parapsychology,* vol. 47, 1983.

86. Described in Jamie McHugh, "Alive at the Edge: Field Notes from an Endangered Species," Internet Paper, 1997.

87. Ibid.

88. Described in HomeArts Network, "Prayer: The Proof," *Country Living's Healthy Living,* Hearst, 1997.

89. Jon Kabat-Zinn, *Full Catastrophe Living: Using the Wisdom of Your Body and Mind to Face Stress, Pain, and Illness,* (New York: Delacorte Press, 1990).

90. E. Laszlo, "Subtle Connections: Psi, Grof, Jung, and the Quantum Vacuum," the International Society of the Systems Sciences and the Club of Budapest, Internet Paper, 1996.

CHAPTER TWO Herbs: Our Green Relatives

1. R. McCaleb, "Boosting Immunity with Herbs," Herb Research Fund website, 1997.
2. Ibid.
3. Ibid.
4. H. Yunde, *Chinese Medical Journal,* 94(1), pp. 35–40, 1981.

CHAPTER FIVE Aromatherapy: The Sweet Breathing of Flowers

1. Valnet, Jean, M.D., *The Practice of Aromatherapy,* (New York: Destiny Books, 1980).
2. Ibid.
3. Pierro Dolara et al., "Analgesis effects of myrrh," *Nature,* vol. 379, p. 29, January 4, 1996.
4. *Chicago Daily Herald,* June 28, 1995.
5. M. Kirk-Smith, P. Parsons, M. Farrell, "Conference Reports," *International Journal of Aromatherapy,* vol. 6, no. 4, pp. 3–5.
6. Ibid.
7. E. N. Frankel et al., "Evaluation of Antioxidant Activity of Rosemary Extracts, Carnosol, and Carnosic Acid on Bulk Vegetable Oils and Fish Oil and Their Emulsions," *Journal of the Science of Food and Agriculture,* vol. 72, no. 2, 1996.
8. M. Kirk-Smith, P. Parsons, M. Farrell, "Conference Reports," *International Journal of Aromatherapy,* vol. 6, no. 4, pp. 3–5.
9. C. Dunn, J. Sleep, D. Collett, "Sensing an Improvement: An Experimental Study to Evaluate the Use of Aromatherapy, Massage and Periods of Rest in an Intensive Care Unit," *Journal of Advanced Nursing,* 21 (1): 34–40, January 1995.
10. A. M. Boyle, J. C. Santelli, "The Effect of Environmental Fragrancing on Patient Anxiety," *The Aromatic Thymes,* vol. 4, no. 1, pp. 35–37, March 1996.
11. Described in *Amanda Arlington, Strategic Health Review,* September 16, 1997.
12. "The Key Role of Smell in an Infant's Bonding, *New York Times,* April 23, 1991, Science Watch.
13. Described in B. Nielsen, Connect, South Carolina Department of Education Website, May 1997.
14. Tiffany M. Field et al., "Stress and Coping in Infancy and Childhood," University of Miami Symposia, vol. 4, 1991.
15. Ibid.
16. C. J. Stevenson, "The Psychophysiological Effects of Aromatherapy Massage Following Cardiac Surgery," *Complementary Therapies in Medicine,* 2(1): 27–35, January 1994.
17. B. Evans, "Nursing: An audit into the effects of aromatherapy massage and the cancer patient in palliative and terminal care," *Complementary Therapies in Medicine,* 3(4): 239–241, October 1995.
18. Jean Valnet, M.D., *The Practice of Aromatherapy,* (New York: Destiny Books, 1980).
19. M. Kirk-Smith, P. Parsons, M. Farrell, "Conference Reports," *International Journal of Aromatherapy,* vol. 6, no. 4, pp. 3–5.

CHAPTER NINE Mother Earth's Guide to Common Ailments

1. Described in: R. E. Vatz and L. E. Weinberg, "Hyperactivity?" *Mothering,* no. 74, Spring 1995.
2. Ibid.
3. Ibid.
4. Randi Henderson, "Relying on Ritalin," *Common Boundary,* vol. 14, issue 3, May/June 1996.

BIBLIOGRAPHY

Armitage, George T. *Ghost Dog and Other Hawaiian Legends*. Honolulu, Hawaii: Advertiser, 1944.

Arnos, Kathy. *Bach Flowers for Children*. Woodbridge, Va.: Discount Newsletter Printing, 1992.

Bach, Edward. *Heal Thyself*. Santa Fe: Sun Books, 1985.

————. *The Twelve Healers and Other Remedies*. London: C. W. Daniel Co. Ltd., 1975.

Barnard, Julian and Martine. *The Healing Herbs of Edward Bach*. Bath, England: Ashgrove Press Ltd., 1994.

Biser, Sam. *Cures from the Last-Chance Clinic*. Charlottesville, Va.: The University of Natural Healing, 1995.

Boericke, William. *Materia Medica with Repertory,* 9th ed. Santa Rosa, Calif.: Boericke and Tafel Inc., 1927.

Bremness, Lesley. *The Complete Book of Herbs*. London: Viking Studio Books, 1988.

Burton Goldberg Group. *Alternative Medicine*. Fife, Wash.: Future Medicine Publishing Inc., 1995.

Callinan, Paul. *Family Homeopathy*. New Canaan, Conn.: Keats Publishing, Inc., 1995.

Crook, William G. *Hyperactivity*. Jackson, Tenn.: Professional Books, 1991.

Curtis, Susan, and Romy Fraser. *Natural Healing for Women*. London: Pandora Press, 1991.

Dadd, Debra Lynn. *Nontoxic, Natural, and Earthwise*. Los Angeles: Jeremey P. Tarcher Inc., 1990.

Davis, Patricia. *Aromatherapy: An A–Z*. Essex, England: C. W. Daniel Co. Ltd., 1988.

Duncan, Alice, and D. C. Likowski. *Your Healthy Child*. Neskowin, Ore.: Sanicula Press, 1995.

Fellner, Tara. *Aromatherapy for You and Your Child*. Boston: Charles E. Tuttle Co. Inc., 1995.

Foley, Daniel J. *Herbs for Use and for Delight*. New York: Dover Publications Inc., 1974.

Frazier, Gregory and Beverly. *The Bath Book*. San Francisco: Troubador Press, 1973.

Gibson, D. M. *Elements of Homeopathy*. New Delhi, India: B. Jain Publishers Pvt. Ltd., 1992.

Hahnemann, Samuel. *Organon of Medicine*. New Delhi, India: B. Jain Publishers, 1995.

Lavabre, Marcel. *Aromatherapy Workbook*. Rochester, Vt.: Healing Arts Press, 1990.

LeBoyer, Frederick. *Loving Hands*. New York: Alfred A. Knopf, 1981.

Lima, Patrick. *The Harrowsmith Book of Herbs*. Ontario, Canada: Camden House Publishing Inc., 1986.

MacFarlane, Ruth B. *Collecting and Preserving Plants*. New York: Dover Publications Inc., 1994.

Montagu, Ashley. *Touching: The Human Significance of the Skin*. New York: Harper and Row, 1986.

Padus, Emrika. *The Complete Guide to Your Emotions and Your Health.* Emmaus, Penn.: Rodale Press, 1986.

Ramsey, Teresa Kirkpatrick. *Baby's First Massage Instructor's Manual.* Centreville, Ohio: self-published, 1995.

Restak, Richard. *The Brain.* New York: Bantam Books, 1984.

Schoemaker, Joyce M., and Charity Y. Vitale. *Healthy Homes, Healthy Kids: Protecting Your Children From Everyday Environmental Hazards.* Washington, D.C.: Island Press, 1991.

Scott, Julian. *Natural Medicine for Children.* New York: Avon Books, 1990.

Sheehan, Kathryn, and Mary Waidner. *Earthchild.* Tulsa, Okla.: Council Oak Books, 1991.

Siegel, Bernie. *Love, Medicine, and Miracles.* New York: Harper and Row, 1986.

Steadman, Alice. *Who's the Matter with Me?* Marina del Rey, Calif.: Devorss and Company, 1966.

Taylor, Richard. *Beeswax Molding and Candlemaking.* Interlaken, N.Y.: Linden Books, 1984.

Tenney, Louise. *Today's Herbal Health for Children.* Pleasant Grove, Utah: Woodland Publishing, 1996.

———. *Today's Herbal Health.* Provo, Utah: Woodland Books, 1983.

Ullman, Dana. *Homeopathic Medicine for Children and Infants.* New York: Tarcher/Putnam, 1992.

Valnet, Jean. *The Practice of Aromatherapy.* New York: Destiny Books, 1980.

Verny, Thomas. *The Secret Life of the Unborn Child.* New York: Summit Books, 1981.

Weatherford, Jack. *Indian Givers.* New York: Fawcett Columbine, 1988.

Weeks, Nora. *The Medical Discoveries of Edward Bach, Physician.* New Canaan, Conn.: Keats Publishing Inc., 1994.

Westland, Pamela. *The Herb Handbook.* New York: Gallery Books, 1991.

FURTHER READING

Bach, Edward. *Heal Thyself.* Santa Fe: Sun Books, 1988.

Barnard, Julian and Martine. *The Healing Herbs of Edward Bach.* Bath: Ashgrove Press, 1995.

Borysenko, Joan, and Miroslav Borysenko. *The Power of the Mind to Heal.* Carson, Calif.: Hay House Inc., 1994.

The Burton Goldberg Group. *Alternative Medicine.* Fife, Wash.: Future Medicine Publishing, Inc., 1995.

Campion, Kitty. *Holistic Woman's Herbal.* Boston: Charles E. Tuttle Co., Inc., 1996.

Childre, Doc Lew. *Teaching Children to Love: 80 Games and Fun Activities for Raising Balanced Children in Unbalanced Times.* Boulder Creek, Calif.: Planetary Publications, 1996.

Colburn, Theo et al. *Our Stolen Future: Are We Threatening Our Fertility, Intelligence, and Survival?* New York: Dutton, 1996.

Dethlefsen, Thorwald, and Rudiger Dahlke. *The Healing Power of Illness: The Meaning of Symptoms and How to Interpret Them.* Dorset: Element Books, 1990.

Dossey, Larry. *Healing Words, The Power of Prayer and the Practice of Medicine.* San Francisco: Harper, 1996.

Fagin, Dan, and Marianne Lavelle. *Toxic Deception.* Secaucus, N.J.: Birch Lane Press, 1997.

Garrett, Laurie. *The Coming Plague: Newly Emerging Diseases in a World Out of Balance.* New York: Penguin, 1996.

Hay, Louise. *You Can Heal Your Life.* Carson, Calif.: Hay House, Inc., 1987.

Montagu, Ashley. *Touching: The Human Significance of the Skin.* New York: Harper and Row, 1986.

Pelletier, Kenneth R. *Mind as Healer, Mind as Slayer.* New York: Delta Books, 1977.

Pipher, Mary. *Reviving Ophelia: Saving the Selves of Adolescent Girls.* New York: Ballantine Books, 1994.

Roads, Michael J. *Talking with Nature.* Tiburon, Calif.: H. J. Kramer, Inc., 1987.

Scott, Julian. *Natural Medicine for Children.* New York: Avon Books, 1990.

Siegel, Bernie. *Love, Medicine, and Miracles: Lessons Learned about Self-Healing from a Surgeon's Experience with Exceptional Patients.* New York: Harper and Row, 1986.

Taylor, Louise, and Lisa Marie Nelson. *The Healthy Family Handbook.* Boston: Charles E. Tuttle Co., Inc., 1997.

Tierra, Michael. *The Way of Herbs.* New York: Pocket Books, 1983.

INDEX

AFTERWORD

This is now a time to weigh the choices for our future. We do have a choice. Nature, the First People, and the spirits of our ancestors are giving you loud warnings. You see increasing floods, more damaging hurricanes, hail storms, climate changes and earthquakes as our prophesies said would come. Even animals and birds are warning us with strange changes in their behavior such as the beaching of whales. Why do animals act like they know about the earth's problems and most humans act like they know nothing?

If we return to spiritual harmony and live from our hearts, we can experience a paradise in this world. It's up to all of us, as children of Mother Earth, to clean up this mess before it's too late.

—Thomas Banyaca, Hopi Elder, Address to the United Nations General Assembly, New York, December 10, 1992